TO:

FROM:

DATE:

KETO K.I.S.S.
Keeping It Super Simple!
Embracing the Keto Lifestyle Journey
By Angie Gleason, RN and Bev Walker,
ISBN: 978-1-7333223-0-0

Published by: The Lifestyle Changers

Medical Disclaimer

The content presented in this book is for the reader's informational and educational purposes only. It is not intended to diagnose or take the place of medical advice or treatment from your personal physician. The information in this book has not been evaluated by the U.S. Food and Drug Administration and is not intended to diagnose, treat, cure or prevent any disease. All readers are advised to consult with qualified medical professionals regarding diet, weight loss, exercise and overall health concerns. Personal physicians should be informed of all nutritional changes. Patients should never stop taking or adjust any medications without consultation of their physician. You are responsible for your own health.

The authors claim no responsibility to any person or entity for any liability, loss, or damage caused by or alleged to be caused directly or indirectly, as a result of the use, application or interpretation of the information presented in this book. While the authors provide information in this book with the desire to help improve overall health, multiple factors may influence results and individual results may vary. Every effort has been made by the authors to ensure the content of this book is accurate, helpful, simple and understandable. This is not in any way an exhaustive coverage of the subject.

Visit www.ketokisslifestyle.com to purchase additional copies

Layout and Cover Art by Bev Walker

Cover Photograph by Abby Shadle
www.abbyshadle.com

First Printing September 2019 / Printed in the United States of America

KETO K.I.S.S.

Keeping It Super Simple!

Embracing the KETO Lifestyle Journey

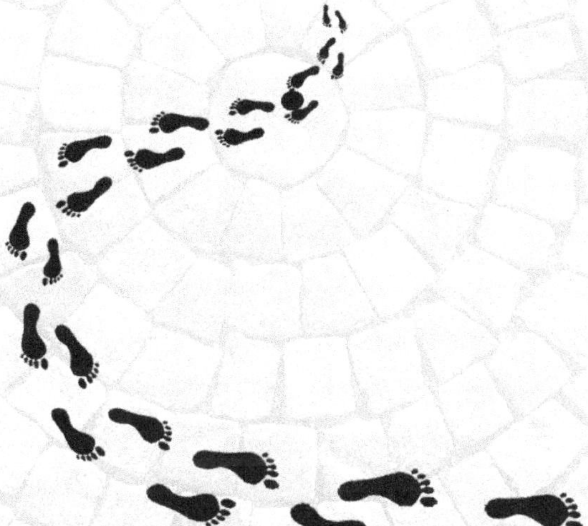

Angie Gleason, RN
Bev Walker

CONTENTS

INTRODUCTION

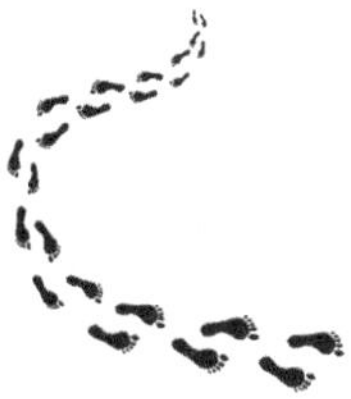

The word "Keto" is causing quite the buzz these days. There is so much information out there on this hot topic! The ketogenic "diet" and this way of eating can be incredibly hard and confusing. This book was written to help you sort through fact and fiction. The Keto lifestyle really is SUPER SIMPLE! You may be thinking that Keto is just a diet. Nope, it's not! We're going to make a very bold statement right here at the beginning:

~ THE KETO LIFESTYLE JOURNEY
CAN CHANGE YOUR LIFE IN MIRACULOUS WAYS! ~

It's a journey that will take you to a place of wellness that you never thought possible! We're pretty sure if you're like us and most people, you probably have various health issues and some of them may be pretty serious. You may have tried a lot of different ways to lose weight and have spent hundreds, if not thousands of dollars on numerous weight loss programs, diets, foods, clinics, coaches or may have even had bariatric surgical procedures. You may just be sick and tired of being sick and tired. Whatever your past experiences, we've got great news!

~ THIS BOOK HAS BEEN WRITTEN JUST FOR YOU! ~

Keto is a super simple lifestyle that starts with a MINDSET. The journey starts with you making a decision that you no longer want to stay where you are. Only you can make that decision. Yes, the results can be really incredible, and we promise you'll find out in this book just how simple this lifestyle is but, IT IS A LIFESTYLE CHANGE. Ok, you just read the word "change". If you're like us, that word may not be one of your favorites. Even though the word "change" sometimes seems intimidating, you will learn and discover things about this lifestyle that are going to be both surprising and amazing. Think of this journey as a commitment to your health and wellness for the rest of your life. It really is a gift you're giving yourself that's truly priceless. While you are making this commitment to yourself, we are making a commitment to you to make this lifestyle change SUPER SIMPLE, very doable and if you can believe it, FUN!

The Keto K.I.S.S. book has a companion journal to stay on course and track your progress. The journal is something we are passionate about. You'll not only be able to stay on track, but you'll be able to look back on how far you've come. When we look back, we still marvel at the remarkable, miraculous changes that have taken place in our lives and our health. We are really excited to address emotions, feelings and how to deal with that aspect of the Keto lifestyle. Let's be real. Emotions and feelings play a MAJOR role when we make lifestyle changes. We're pretty sure this is the only Keto book and journal that actually talks about the emotional mindset and offers proven solutions. An important and cool thing about this book and journal is you are going to have links to a huge community of fellow Keto'ers that are also on this journey! Our Keto community of friends will be there to support, encourage, cheer you on and help you celebrate all the crazy, wonderful results you're going to see. You will find that it is so much more fun and enjoyable if you don't Keto alone! So, come and join us, The Lifestyle Changers, on this extraordinary Keto lifestyle journey. Adventure and astonishing results await you!

OUR STORIES

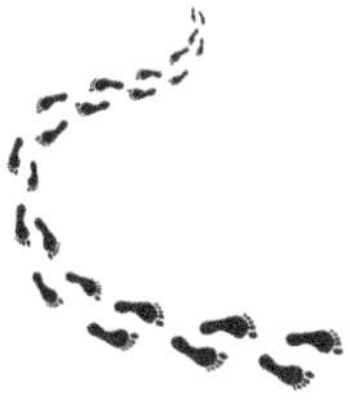

Stories are super powerful and so important to share. Miracles have happened in our lives and we cannot keep quiet! We tell our stories to inspire and encourage you and to show that this lifestyle is not always easy but definitely simple. We openly share our struggles and victories. We believe that sharing our triumphs as well as our struggles has incredible potential for you to see how this same Keto journey can transform your life, too. We share our testimonies with the hope and prayer that many lives will be forever changed! We celebrate how differently God has created us and bonded our lives together to bring you the Keto K.I.S.S. book and journal. We wholeheartedly agree that we are divinely created and everything we go through in our lives is for a purpose. By telling our stories we're loaning our faith to you so you can know in your heart that God CAN heal you on this amazing journey! Our stories are very different as you will see. We have come from completely different starting points, but God has merged our paths together on this Keto lifestyle journey. We begin with our stories...

ANGIE'S STORY

I knew without a doubt I was destined to become a nurse. I got my calling at the age of 14 when God miraculously spared my life after my appendix ruptured. I marveled at the love and care I got from doctors and nurses over the 2 months of hospitalizations and 2 major surgeries I had. I knew for sure in my heart that that's what I wanted to do for the rest of my life…love and care for people. It really is a calling for sure! I went straight from high school into nursing school and at the age of 19 I was working in a hospital as a LPN. I got married at age 21, went back to college and became a RN. My nursing career has spanned over 41 years. Yes, that's a crazy long time!

Through the years it was very obvious that despite our advanced technology and medical practices, people were getting sicker and sicker and more and more dis-eases were coming onto the scene. (I spelled dis-ease that way on purpose after all it is DIS-EASE!) The truth is: WE DON'T HAVE A HEALTHCARE SYSTEM. WE HAVE A DIS-EASE MANAGEMENT SYSTEM! I'm sure you can agree with that statement. As a nurse who was called to care for, teach and help heal and restore health, this really breaks my heart. I went into nursing to see people get well and live happy, healthy lives. Could these conditions be prevented? If so, then how? If medications, pills and potions really worked, you wouldn't need a prescription refill, right? Stop and think about that. I can assure you these are the things I've pondered.

Let me set the stage a bit to let you know where I'm coming from with my Keto lifestyle. I'm a 60 year old, post-menopausal, Type 1 Diabetic (T1D). My pancreas does not make insulin at all. I have an insulin pump that I use to deliver my insulin to me. I control as best I can what a person's pancreas does normally for them. This diagnosis makes my Keto lifestyle journey unique and very challenging at times but I'm living proof that it's TOTALLY DOABLE! I discovered early on how to make Keto SUPER SIMPLE so, here I am sharing with you so you can discover how amazingly SIMPLE it really is. The way I figure, the simpler it is, the easier it will be for your lifestyle change and the sweeter (pun intended) your success will be.

I was diagnosed with gestational diabetes at age 35 with my 4th baby and after his birth my pancreas stopped making insulin. After I was diagnosed with T1D I thought I had it all figured out with my medical knowledge as a RN and handled my diabetes care mostly on my own. Please note: I do not advise that at all! If you have diabetes, please work with your doctor and do your own research. This journey has not been easy, but it certainly has been fascinating, sometimes frustrating but overall a fun adventure. I never dreamed I'd be sharing my incredible story but honestly, I can't keep quiet! So, here's how I discovered the Keto lifestyle....

I've struggled with being overweight all my life even as a child. I've been on just about every weight loss program there is, spent lots of money on expensive pills and potions and wasted time and money on gym memberships and exercise equipment. Do you feel me?? Yeah, I lost a little weight here and there, but it usually packed right back on plus some. I'm guessing you have a similar story. Sadly, most of us do, right?

Here's the kicker, as a diabetic with an insulin pump I soon found out that I could eat anything my heart desired. I could be "normal". All I had to do was figure out how much insulin I needed for the amount of carbs in the food I wanted to eat. Cheesecake, ice cream, potatoes, bread, no problem! I could have it all! There was a big problem with that though. I'd guesstimate without measuring and give myself insulin which sent me on a blood sugar rollercoaster with super high and super low blood sugars. I assure you that rollercoasters are only fun at amusement parks. Of course, I was setting myself up for major complications and this was very dangerous way to live. I felt horrible and I gained a lot more weight to my already overweight body in the process. I was pretty mortified that I was considered morbidly obese (it said so on my chart at the doctor's office). My final breaking point came at the age of 58. I topped the scale at the weight I swore to myself I'd never get to. I'm 5'2" and tipped the scale at 205 pounds!! The world was telling me to be happy with who I was. I had come to the conclusion to just embrace and enjoy my life. I really tried even though I was completely miserable. How can you enjoy life when you're sick, depressed and overwhelmed with stress? There were some days I just couldn't even get out of bed. I had all kinds of aches and pains, got sick easily due to a compromised immune system, had headaches on a daily basis, etc. Depression set in big time, but I became super good at hiding it. Hiding depression became a full time job. I got to the point where I just accepted that my destiny was to eventually suffer the complications of diabetes and succumb to the disease that took my daddy's life at age 63. Looking back, that scares me. I remember how devastating it was to see my daddy try so hard to keep his type 1 diabetes under control. It makes me both sad and angry that we did not know about the Keto lifestyle back then! He followed the American Diabetes Associations diet (for the most part), had kidney failure, dialysis, got a kidney transplant, had amputations and was legally blind when he died at 63 years of age. I just turned 60 years old at the writing of this book. This seriously makes my heart hurt.

Ok, let's change gears and fast forward to 2014. I discovered the world of natural health and essential oils. I started teaching health and wellness classes but there was one huge problem. Me! I was HUGE. How could anyone take me seriously? All people had to do was look at me and see that I was not healthy. You just can't camouflage your extra poundage. That's when I decided to get serious about my health and weight.

I expressed my desire to lose weight and get my blood sugars under better control with my endocrinologist. She sent me to a diabetes dietician to help me "fix" my out of control blood sugars and hopefully shed some of the weight I'd accumulated. The dietician lectured me on what I had already known to follow. You know, the American Diabetes Associations (ADA) Diet which is pretty much the Standard American Diet (SAD). Her instructions to me as a T1D was to eat 3 meals a day consisting of at least 45 grams of carbs per meal and at least 2 snacks a day consisting of 15 grams of carbs each. WHAT??!! That's 165 grams of carbs a day for a person who can't metabolize carbs!! You're going to find out in this book how INSANE that is! I asked her about the Keto diet that my son-in-law had been on with great success and she got the look of horror on her face. She told me I'd end up in ICU on a ventilator if I did that! Of course, she was confusing ketosis with ketoacidosis, a life threatening condition that people with T1D can experience with very high blood sugars. Her response triggered a rebel-spirited response in me saying, "Oh heck no! This can't be right!" I set out to prove her wrong because for the past 25 years the American Diabetes Associations Diet did not work for me or any other diabetic that I knew of. There had to be something I was missing, right??

So, this was the beginning of my Keto lifestyle journey. I was really surprised at what I learned! While doing my research, believe me I did a lot of that, I decided to start out slow by just simply eliminating everything white from my diet. That included rice, bread, pasta and potatoes. These things are the most damaging carbs you can consume. Eliminating them was the hardest part starting out that I faced hands down! I had to check my blood sugar every few hours and adjust my insulin which was pretty difficult to do without guidance. I felt like I was N=1 in my own research experiment. (N=1...that's when you are the only one in the study being done.) I felt like I was all alone, but I knew in my heart that it was something I had to do. It was a bit scary too, I must admit but I was very determined. (**Let me say again, if you have been diagnosed with type 1 or 2 diabetes and are on medications please do not do this without the care of your doctor.**) As I did my research, I watched videos and read articles that gave me so many different emotions on this new journey that I was embarking on. I was excited, hopeful and sometimes just plain giddy. On the other hand, I became very angry and frustrated at all the LIES I had been told by my doctors and my anger even went back to the lies I had been taught in nursing school! One question that really haunted me was if my T1D daddy had lived this Keto lifestyle, would he still be alive today? Like I said before, that question hurts my heart big time! Consider this as me shouting...The Standard American Diet (SAD) and the food pyramid are WRONG!! Flat out WRONG! WE'VE BEEN LIED TO!

I started my Keto lifestyle journey in April of 2017 at the age of 58.

Yes, a 58 year old post-menopausal T1D mama of 5 adult kiddos just changed her life.... completely! Crazy, huh? I started out and never looked back. Ok, truth is, I did look back but only at my "before" photos and measurements. I can hardly believe I ever looked like that or measured that big. I sometimes cry and shudder to think where I would be now if I had not started this journey. I can honestly say I never dreamed I'd have the results and testimony that I have and certainly never dreamed I'd be writing a book but here I am! I feel better at 60 than I did in my 30's! I've gone from a size 16/18 jeans to a size 4/6, size 2x top to a small/medium and have lost almost 70 pounds and over 84 inches! My A1c (lab value for 3 month average of blood sugars) went from a high 8.0 to a normal 5.4! Needless to say, I never went back to that diabetes dietician and my new endocrinologist is super happy and encouraging. Hallelujah!

I'm so glad you're embarking on this journey too! I want you to know I've prayed over this book and specifically for all the people that will have their lives changed in miraculous ways...that's YOU! I'm excited for you and cannot wait to hear your story! It's going to be AMAZING!

Blessings,
Angie

BEV'S STORY

I never would have believed I would be writing about the struggles and triumphs of my weight loss journey. God had a reason for each step of the road I have walked. He has led me to a lifestyle that is bringing about incredible health results, self-discipline that I did not think possible and major personal growth in my life. This journey led me to co-authoring this book and it is a story that God has clearly said must be shared.

My personality type is an extreme introvert. Being in crowds literally wears me out and I cherish my alone time! I'm a very logical thinker and tend to stay in my head and keep my heart and feelings tucked away. For me to be sharing any of this with you is just short of a miracle...one that God is performing every step of the way while I'm writing this.

Food has been my comfort, my silent friend, my way to celebrate, my reward system and my downfall for years. Some of the old messages that have played in my mind since childhood are:

"You are supposed to be perfect."
"Food is your emotional support."
"Food is your comfort."
"Children are to be seen and not heard."

I have struggled with my weight from the time I turned 6 after I had my tonsils out. I don't think I could eat much before that because I had constant sore throats and ear infections, but my habit was to eat food when I needed comforting and I certainly did that! In my teens I did a well-known weight loss program that's initials are WW off and on and it helped keep the weight down for a short period of time.

Before I got married, I managed to lose weight and look great for our wedding! Two years later we had our first daughter. While I was pregnant with her, I told myself I could eat anything I wanted. I had a 70 pound weight gain and was diagnosed with gestational diabetes. Some of the weight came off after I delivered but the majority stayed intact. My weight just crept higher and higher each year. Of course, during this time I tried every fad diet that came along only to lose and then gain back more than I had lost. Eight years later our 2nd daughter was born, and I weighed 260. I quit getting on the scales because I didn't want to know what they said. I remember weighing once and I weighed 319! I did not get on the scales after that for years.

In 2006 my primary care physician asked me if I had ever thought about having bariatric lap band surgery. At that point I had been diagnosed with type 2 diabetes and was on prescription meds to control it. I weighed 263 when I had the surgery and I got down to 170 in the year that followed.

My diabetes was gone, and I no longer had to take the meds for it. I was able to maintain my weight loss for 9 years and then something happened. I had heartburn all the time and pain from my port. I started drinking milk shakes and gained about 15 pounds. I went to see my surgeon and he suggested taking the lap band out and doing a gastric sleeve procedure.

At this point I didn't think I had much of a choice. I was so miserable. Unfortunately, the surgery got postponed and I didn't have it for 2 more months. I continued to gain weight for a total of about 35 pounds before my lap band removal/gastric sleeve procedure. I had no energy, tired all the time, grumpy and ready for the surgery that I thought was going to fix it all for good. What I didn't realize at that time was my blood sugar was creeping back up and most likely my type 2 diabetes was back. I didn't even think about checking into it at the time. The surgery went well, and I lost about 15 pounds quickly, but things slowed down significantly.

A year after my surgery I had my blood sugar drawn as part of a program at work and it was 165, which is very high for a fasting count. I knew it was high but ignored it and did nothing about it. The next year I participated again in this program and guess what?? My fasting blood sugar was nearly identical… ok, wakeup call! This time I slowly started really trying to cut out the obvious sugar in my diet but not really cutting out foods that contained a lot of carbs. I monitored my fasting blood sugar levels here and there and it was ranging between 125 – 150. It was improving but by no means where it should have been.

In April 2017 my friend Angie started the Keto lifestyle. I watched her results and progress. I was totally amazed at the transformation in her! We went to hear a chiropractor friend speak one evening about changing habits. He said that the mind and body need 66 days to truly change a habit. As I left that night, I told Angie I was going to commit to the Keto lifestyle for the next 66 days to see what would happen. Guess what? It was amazing! I felt so much better and inches seemed to be melting off (I forgot to measure the first day). The scales truly didn't move that much. I ended up losing 12 pounds early on which was awesome because to that point the surgery had really not helped me to lose any.

I am not going to lie to you. Those first 4 weeks on my Keto journey were not easy. Following the Keto lifestyle is simple but not always easy. I still had an emotional attachment to the comfort foods I loved. Giving those up was hard but I was determined. Here's the thing though, I felt better than I had in a really long time! My clothes were fitting differently so I knew my body was changing but in my mind I struggled because the scale wasn't moving. Even with the positive changes I was experiencing like more energy and better focus, I still fought with my emotions and the stronghold food had on me.

A few months later discouragement got the best of me and I fell completely off the Keto lifestyle path. At this point, it was closing in on the holidays and I just said forget it because this Keto life wasn't working for me anyway! Slowly I went back to my old habits listening to the messages stuck in my head that had always led to failure in the past. I was feeling totally lethargic, eating anything and everything I wanted, and I felt terrible! During those 2 months my blood sugar crept way up, the inflammation in my joints that had improved so much was now back to continual pain and I was quickly regaining the weight I had lost.

I knew I had to make a change in the upcoming new year, so I EMOTIONALLY prepared myself for making a PERMANENT LIFESTYLE CHANGE for my health. I felt a total difference in my body being back on sugar and carbs and it was an eye-opening experience after not eating them for so long. I could not deny it any longer. My body cannot handle sugar and carbs! I am truly insulin resistant!

Over the last 8 months my body has been in healing mode and has responded incredibly well to the Keto lifestyle. My A1c 3 years ago was 7.0 which was way above normal range. My recent A1c was 5.0 – NORMAL! If there is one thing I want you to hear from me it is this, **DON'T GIVE UP**, **TRUST THE PROCESS**! I damaged my body for so many years with the foods that I indulged in and it is taking time for it to heal.

God has put us on this KETO lifestyle journey for a reason and has placed it in both of our hearts to share our stories and write this book. We believe that this is only the beginning of this adventure and it certainly is constantly evolving! We have experienced so many "God moments" it has been amazing beyond words! What I do want you to know is that this book is from God to you! I know that with every part of my being! He has led me down the path I have been on for the last 60 years to be able to share it with you and now He wants to use the Keto K.I.S.S. book and journal/planner to truly transform your health and wellness both EMOTIONALLY and PHYSICALLY. We want this to be a journey that we take together. This book and journal are just the first steps to your new lifestyle. We will be with you all along the way using social media posts, videos and live interactions to stay connected and support each other. Our prayer is that your life is changed in unimaginable ways!

Prayers & Hugs,
Bev

CHAPTER 1

Getting Ready for Your Keto Lifestyle Journey

Every journey you'll ever take in your life starts with deciding where you want to go, planning your path and then taking that very first exciting, maybe daring and sometimes scary step into uncharted territory. Trying to embark out on your own can make things kind of difficult. What if you could have tour guides who have experienced some really amazing things on this same journey you are about to set out on? What if you could avoid the roadblocks, detours and treacherous off-roading that could throw you off course? This book will serve as your personal planning guide and help you navigate this crazy, fun adventure all along the way!

Benefits of the Keto Lifestyle

First, let's look at a few of the HUGE BENEFITS this lifestyle includes. Most of us begin the Keto lifestyle to lose weight, not even realizing the miraculous impact that this journey can have on our health and wellness.

Countless testimonies show the benefits of the Keto lifestyle include:

- Weight loss…LOTS of it
- May reverse Type 2 Diabetes
- Blood sugar balance, stops insulin resistance
- Supports healthy brain function, clears brain fog, increases cognition and focus
- Treats/prevents neurological disorders like Alzheimer's, Parkinson's and Dementia
- Healthy gut, no bloating, no reflux, no heartburn
- Improves or gets rid of Irritable Bowel Syndrome, Colitis, Crohn's Disease
- Decreases generalized inflammation
- Reverses fatty liver and pancreas
- Decreases chronic pain including migraines
- Increases energy and endurance
- Improves/prevents fibromyalgia
- Balances hormones…all of them
- Epilepsy treatment
- Improves mood
- Improves and/or gets rid of ADHD and ADD
- Improves sleep and sleeping disorders
- Decreases depression, anxiety, PTSD
- Eliminates skin issues like acne, eczema and psoriasis
- Improves/manages/clears up arthritis
- Improves fertility, PCOS
- Slows the aging process
- Starves cancer cells

Oh my goodness! It is so exciting to think of how these benefits could totally change your life or the life of your loved ones! The thought of the changes that could take place in someone's life makes this a very emotional subject for us! When looking at all these major benefits there is a huge, key factor, OUR GUT HEALTH! We don't want you to miss this about the Keto lifestyle. Much of our overall health depends on our gut and what we feed it. If we consumed the foods and nutrients our bodies were designed to eat, we would prevent a great percentage of these dis-eases from ever happening! Yes, "dis-ease" is spelled like that for a reason. After all, it's not the "ease" or state of wellness our bodies were designed to function in. Our bodies were created to consume specific foods for optimal health.

The great news is you can improve, manage or cure many health issues simply by changing what foods you eat. Unfortunately, the truth is, sometimes it takes a really horrible health crisis to get people's attention. The first thing we do is run to the doctor, have all kinds of tests done and get a diagnosis. Then there's always a pill or treatment plan to manage the symptoms never discussing nutrition or lifestyle changes to improve or cure the dis-ease! Doctors and nurses have little to no education on nutrition in medical or nursing school. What little they do get is the Standard American Diet food pyramid and information based on LIES. Yes, these are lies and that is a strong word. The whole food pyramid should be turned completely upside down with the fats on the bottom, proteins in the middle and carbohydrates on the top! We highly encourage you to do your own research as you read this book and learn about the Keto lifestyle. It's your life and health we're talking about here! It's so important! We cannot stress that enough!

CHAPTER 2

KETO is NOT a DIET, It's a LIFESTYLE!

The Keto lifestyle is not a new fad! Our ancestors as far back as we can go before modern times lived this way. Think about that. The only time they consumed fruits and vegetables were when they were in season which was maybe 1 to 2 months out of the year depending on where they lived. They lived off of fats and protein the majority of the time from hunting. They ate every part of the animals they hunted. That's the way our bodies were uniquely designed. It's in our DNA. Back in the day there were no processed foods, fast food restaurants, chemically produced artificial ingredients, GMOs or even sugar added to the foods they ate.

Let's be real here from the start with a few truth bombs. There are some things we need to make clear before we get into the simple basics. If you truly expect to benefit from all the awesome things Keto can accomplish in your life and body, it has to become your new

LIFESTYLE. Please hear us out! It's not some magical thing you do for a little while and go back to the place where you started this journey... For some, it may have taken months or years to make the decision to turn your life in a new direction and learn what Keto is all about. Now you have this book in your hands and have read to this point… if you are still on the fence, IT IS DECISION TIME!

There are a couple things you really need to consider, carb addiction and your mindset. Did you know that sugar is more addictive than cocaine? It's true! Research and studies prove this fact. We understand this struggle all too well in fact, we still struggle at times and have discovered amazing ways to handle this part of the journey. That's why we decided to address the emotional and psychological part of this journey as well as how to overcome this mental stronghold that food has over us. It's like the proverbial "elephant in the room" that no other Keto book will address.

Here's a question to ask yourself… What is your motivation or your "why" for embarking on this journey? The more intense your reason for this lifestyle change, the more motivated you'll be. The more motivated you are, the faster you'll see changes and results which will excite you to stay on your journey. We can promise you that once you take off on this new road you'll not want to go back! We are pretty sure that most people that start this journey do it because of the weight loss benefit. We really want to emphasize that the benefits to your long term health far outweigh (pun intended!) the exciting weight loss goals you have in mind.

Before you embark on any journey in life you need to know where you're going and how to get there, right? It's the same with this Keto lifestyle journey. You may have researched Keto and are pretty familiar with it or you may have no clue at all about where to start and what all the excitement is about.

Angie: *"I totally understand if you are running around in circles and can't really find a starting point. That was me! My son-in-law had started Keto and I was fascinated with his awesome results but when he shared with me that he was staying at 20 grams of carbs per day, well, that freaked me out! As a type 1 diabetic on an insulin pump I figured that I never could do that because I had been told to follow the American Diabetes Association's recommendation which is actually very high in carbs! I was very intrigued, and my curiosity got the best of me. I had so many questions I needed answered but I really wanted to start ASAP. I heard a friend tell me she had started by eliminating everything white from her diet meaning things like bread, potatoes, pasta and rice. That was the hardest part for me for sure! I was determined to do the 'eliminate everything white' thing while I researched and learned as much as I could about the Keto lifestyle. The really amazing thing was that I saw and felt changes right away!"*

Whether you want to start your journey out slow or go full speed ahead, do what your heart is telling you to do! Either way is ok! The most important thing to remember is to just take that FIRST STEP! You've heard that every journey starts with that first step and we promise once you take it, your whole life is going to change!

Ok, now that we have gotten those things out of the way, come on and let's get on the road!

The more intense your reason for this lifestyle change, the more motivated you will be!

CHAPTER 3

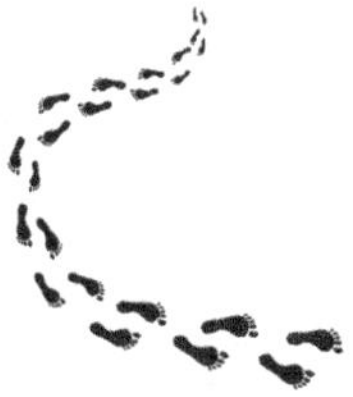

Keto Explained…
Keeping It Super Simple!

Our bodies are divinely, uniquely and wonderfully made by our Creator with the ability to either burn carbohydrates or fat for energy. Crazy, right!? Here's the cool part: YOU HAVE THE POWER TO FLIP THE SWITCH FROM BURNING CARBS TO BURNING FAT! So, let's define Keto. When we say Keto, we're talking about the ketogenic lifestyle or being in the state of ketosis. When you're in ketosis, you are burning fat or ketones as fuel for energy instead of burning carbs (carbohydrates) or sugar for energy.

Here's some scientific, nerdy stuff made simple…Every cell in our bodies have mitochondria. The mitochondria of every cell in our bodies can burn either fat or carbs depending on what we give it. The mitochondria in our cells are responsible for creating 90% of the energy our bodies need to support life and support organ function. Remember studying the parts of the cell in biology class? Here's a little refresher just in case you missed it. The mitochondria are considered the powerhouse or furnace of your cells that turns food into fuel for energy. The goal of the Keto lifestyle is to switch the mitochondria to burn fat (ketones) for energy which it is totally capable of doing. When your body is producing ketones, you will be burning stored fat. That's where the magic begins to take over and amazing things start to happen! You're going to start to feel more energy, think clearer, your discomfort will decrease and inflammation in your body will start to clear up. Plus, you'll notice your clothes fitting differently and you'll have weight loss! Sorry to interject this but it is an important thing to realize. Your cells can only use one type of energy at a time. The kicker is your body will choose carbs over fat for energy every single time. If you eat way more carbs than your body needs for energy, then the excess is stored as your BODY FAT. Bummer, right!? Why is that though? Answer: Insulin.

The goal of the Keto lifestyle is to switch the mitochondria to burn fat (ketones) for energy.

Let's talk about insulin because it plays a huge role here. It's the main hormone that controls your blood sugar and fat storage. It's secreted by the beta cells in your pancreas. We need insulin to survive but out of control insulin secretion in our bodies gets us into a whole lot of trouble! It's really important for you to understand how it all works.

Here you go:

1) You eat carbs (sugar, bread, pasta, cereal, potatoes, rice, etc.).
2) Your body breaks down the carbs immediately into glucose and it gets released into your bloodstream…that's called your blood sugar.
3) Your pancreas releases insulin to get the blood sugar into your cells.
4) The sugar enters the cells and puts your body into carb burning and fat storage mode.

Here's the scoop: To lose weight and burn fat you need to lower your blood sugar and insulin levels. How do you do that?? Answer: By embarking on the Keto lifestyle journey!

There are so many awesome things about burning fat and being in ketosis but a really fascinating fact is that ketones have an antioxidant effect so there are fewer free radicals in our body. What exactly does that mean?? The word antioxidant has been in the spotlight over the last several years, however most people have no idea what the role of an antioxidant really is. Let's simplify it. Antioxidants are substances found in food that stop or delay damage to our cells. They help clean up and remove waste products in your cells called free radicals. Free radicals come from toxins. (we'll discuss toxins a bit later) So, to put it simply, when there are ketones in your body, there's a detoxing, anti-aging effect!

Here's another incredible fact. Studies show that the Keto lifestyle starves cancer cells! Cancer cells get their energy from sugar. The normal, non-cancerous cells in our bodies are able to switch from carb burning to fat burning and are able to use the ketones for energy. Cancer cells can ONLY use glucose (sugar) for energy and growth.

Cancer cells cannot use ketones for energy!

The Keto lifestyle is metabolically very powerful. It controls blood sugar and insulin levels. Research and studies show chronically, sustained high insulin levels due to excessive carb intake is the cause of almost all chronic dis-eases we suffer from. Did you hear that? You might want to read that again and let it sink in! Keto balances both blood sugar and insulin levels to where they need to be.

Let's talk about obesity and stored fat for a moment. You know, we're talking about the fat that's on your belly, butt, thighs and various places stored up because you've been eating too many carbs for so many years. It's stored there just waiting to be used for energy, but we continue to feed our bodies with carbs and those carbs would have to totally be burned for energy before your body could ever get to the stored fat. If you're continually eating carbs there's no reason for that fat to budge and believe us, it won't! As soon as you significantly decrease your carb intake and increase the good fats you eat, your body kicks in and starts burning that stored fat. For real! IT'S REALLY THAT SIMPLE!

Your body either burn carbs or ketones for energy.

You have the power to flip the switch to burn ketones!

CHAPTER 4

Dispelling the Myths, Fallacies and Flat Out Lies

Let's expose some of the huge lies we've been told and have believed. We have each struggled with every single one of these. How in the world has society and even the medical profession gotten away with these things? These are just some facts for you to ponder. You've heard the saying, "Fool me once shame on you. Fool me twice, shame on me", right? Let's not be fooled anymore!

~ **Eating fat makes you fat.** The truth is eating a lot of healthy fats and very low carb helps you BURN fat. We're told to avoid butter, bacon and fatty sources of meats. With the Keto lifestyle you slather butter on everything, cook with it and even put it in your coffee! (More on that in a bit) We were told to only eat lean meats and now we can enjoy good fatty meats like ribeye steaks cooked in bacon grease and dark meat chicken with the skin on, BACON and pork chops. If you are a bacon lover like we both are, you are probably smiling from ear to ear! Good saturated fats do NOT clog your arteries! Eat as much as you want!

~ **We are told that in order to lose weight, we need to count calories.** NOPE. You don't have to count them – ever! Really…not even one! We would like to encourage you to look up the "calories in, calories out" fallacy if you're curious about how all that came to be. The truth is, when you are in ketosis, counting carbs and eating good fats, your body will tell you when it's hungry and when it's satisfied. Maybe for the first time ever in your life you'll learn to listen to what your body is saying to you!

Angie: *"Eating lots of good fat fills me up really fast. Listening to my body's hunger and satisfaction signals has kept me from the heartburn, reflux and digestive issues I suffered from for so many years. When I started listening to my physical cues, I just naturally ate less without worrying and stressing about calories. The freedom and stress relief I have experienced from not having to count calories has made me incredibly happy!"*

Eating fat does
NOT make you fat!

~ **We are told lower our salt intake because that leads to high blood pressure which can lead to heart attacks and strokes.** You guessed it; you do not have to limit your salt intake! Our bodies need salt. The important thing here to note is that not all salt is equal. Table salt is processed and has anti-caking agents… not good! Himalayan pink salt is a great salt to use because of its nutritional value, minerals, electrolytes, and natural iodine. It is a good source of magnesium and promotes a healthy pH level in your body.

~ **We believe we have to have carbs for energy.** Nope! That's not true! Actually, ketones are the ideal clean energy source for your body, especially your brain. When people hear about Keto for the first time most say, "I would die without carbs"! You may THINK you'll die at first, but we promise you won't!! We are both amused and saddened when we hear this statement. It tells us 2 things. First, people don't really understand carbs vs. ketones as an energy source and second, they don't even realize that they are addicted to carbs. The carb addiction thing is super hard to admit and come to grips with. It was for both of us. No one truly wants to admit they are addicted to anything.

~ **We have to eat 3 meals a day.** We're told and taught all our lives that there's breakfast, lunch and dinner and of course we've got to throw in a few snacks here and there, right? Do we REALLY need to do that? No, we don't! The truth is, the result of eating 3 meals a day plus snacks keeps our insulin levels chronically elevated so we do not burn stored fat. (This is where insulin resistance comes in otherwise known as type 2 diabetes.) We burn carbs and the excess carbs we consume turns into more fat. History dispels the three meals a day plus snacks myth. Let's take a look back at the way our ancestors ate once again to help paint the picture. They only ate when food was available, and their diets consisted mostly of animals they had hunted. They had veggies and fruits maybe only 1 to 2 months out of the year when it was in season depending on where they lived. They fasted a lot! (Fasting is an incredible topic we will address in a bit.) Trust us on this, your DNA knows how to do the Keto lifestyle! The 3 meals a day thing goes back to around the industrial time period. Think about the impact on the food industry if we ate 3 meals a day plus snacks! Can you connect the dots? In the 1920's the government intervened, and it all went down the tubes from there. News flash: THERE IS NOTHING IN MEDICAL LITERATURE THAT SAYS EATING 3 MEALS A DAY IS NECESSARY! There is absolutely no research that says that! In fact, there's lots of research and literature on the benefits of fasting.

~ **Living the healthy Keto lifestyle is expensive.** WRONG! The truth is you do not need any pills, powders or potions that doctors or anyone out there are pushing on people. Manufacturers prey on people that are on or fixing to embark on this Keto journey. They market their products "Keto" or "Low Carb" which are really nothing more than processed junk. Just say NO! All you need for your Keto lifestyle can be found at your local grocery store, farmers market, or health food store. For real! In fact, the coolest "secret weapon" of your new lifestyle is absolutely FREE! Can you guess what that is?? Ok, this book is about keeping it super simple so here is the answer.... it's FASTING! Yep.... that's FREE!

~ **Then there's the HUGE cholesterol issue.** Cholesterol will be addressed in the next chapter where fats are discussed. There is a huge fallacy that fats are bad, and cholesterol is the culprit of heart dis-ease and stroke. We'll explain this subject in a little more detail but just know this is not the truth! The perfect storm was created when this lie was perpetrated and profited by both the food industry and big pharma. This is still a major thing in the medical field unfortunately.

CHAPTER 5

Breaking It All Down Into Macronutrients

What in the world is a macronutrient? Let's dive right in because this is super important to know. The Keto lifestyle is basically a very low carb, high fat, moderate protein and whole food way of eating. We'll go into detail about carbs, fat and protein because you'll be tracking them on this journey. These three nutrients are called macronutrients and to keep it simple we're going to call them "macros".

Guess what?? Only 2 of the 3 macros are necessary to sustain your life and health. This was a shock at first!

Can you guess which ones they are by now, right? Ok, here is the scoop. The answer is FAT (lots of it) and PROTEIN (a moderate amount). Surprised? Fact: There are essential fats (fatty acids) and essential proteins (amino acids) but **THERE ARE NO ESSENTIAL**

CARBS! Truth: You can live without carbs! A person can live a healthy life just on lots of good fats and protein.

Let's make this macro thing really simple, ok? There is no need to get hung up, stressed and frustrated on percentages, grams, calories and all the counting and tracking. In the beginning you will want your main focus to be on counting your carbs and keeping them below 20 grams a day as well as ensuring you are eating enough good saturated fats. Ideally, once you get started, you'll discover the information about percentages of each macro, and you will want to track those. Of course, everyone is different and some of you really love math so that information has been included as we talk about each macro. We both have tracked our macros on one of our favorite phone apps called Carb Manager. A word of caution about tracking on apps... Do not let the app tell you what to eat! At the end of the day if you haven't met all your total macros, don't think you have to eat more food. Listen to what your body is telling you, if you aren't hungry, don't eat!

Angie: *"Even though I used an app, for the first whole year of my Keto journey, I really only counted carb grams. Yes! That's it. Just carbs! I counted carbs, ate lots of bacon, eggs, fatty sources of meats and slathered everything in butter! "*

We have provided our Keto Food List in the back of the book for easy reference. It includes all the wonderful foods that you can choose from to create your culinary dishes.

Fats

You'll be eating a lot of healthy fats. In fact, good saturated fats will account for 70-75% of your total daily intake of food. Wow, right? We're sure this surprises most people as it did us in the beginning. All of our lives we have been told eating fats make you fat and is the cause of heart dis-ease and stroke. Adding butter, bacon, good saturated fats and fatty sources of meat may be weird to you at first. Please understand, YOU DO NOT NEED TO FEAR GOOD FATS EVER AGAIN! Increasing your fat intake can take some time to get used to but imagine slathering butter on everything you consume and being able to eat bacon every day! Oh goodness! Your focus should be on making sure you eat enough good, healthy fats every day. Healthy fats fill you up and keep you satisfied for long periods of time, so go ahead and truly enjoy them!

Let's distinguish here between good fats and bad fats. The healthy fats are SATURATED FATS. The very best fats are from natural, organic, grass-fed sources. This includes butter, lard, coconut oil, avocado oil, ghee and bacon grease. One of our favorite oils to use is coconut oil. Make sure and purchase a large jar of coconut oil and get ready for a real treat! You will learn to use it every day by putting it in your coffee and cooking with it.

We would do you a huge disservice if we did not tell you some of the incredibly amazing benefits of MCT oil. MCT stands for medium chain triglycerides which is the BEST saturated fatty acid! Without getting all nerdy on the chemistry and for the sake of keeping it super simple, here are some of the awesome benefits of MCT oil:

- WEIGHT LOSS! MCT oil is processed by the liver and is IMMEDIATELY converted to ketones for energy instead of being stored as fat. This is why MCT oil actually enhances the Keto lifestyle like crazy! It improves thyroid function that aids in metabolism, suppresses your appetite and is shown to have effects similar to intermittent fasting! (We will talk about intermittent fasting coming up soon!)

- It improves energy and endurance as it is easily digested for sustained energy and increased metabolism.
- The ketones created from MCT oil increases memory and brain function and are considered the BEST fuel for your brain.
- It prevents heart disease and high blood pressure through its anti-inflammatory effect in our circulatory systems.
- MCT helps improve digestion and nutrient absorption by balancing your gut micro biome.
- MCT oil is antiviral, antibacterial and anti-fungal!

As we mentioned earlier, coconut oil is one of our favorite oils to use on a daily basis and a really awesome fact about coconut oil is that it contains about 66% MCT oil! Pretty amazing fact, huh?

Fats will account for the greatest percentage of calories you consume. Remember, the really great thing about the Keto lifestyle journey is YOU DON'T HAVE TO COUNT CALORIES! Yep, we shouted that because remember we are all about keeping it super simple! Calorie counting doesn't work anyway because the actual SOURCE of the calories is more important than the AMOUNT of calories you consume. Read that last sentence again. That's crazy great news, right? It can be hard to believe but it is true! Doesn't it just make you so ecstatically happy about not having to count calories? Doesn't that relieve so much stress?? Alleviating as much stress from our lives as we can should be a top priority.

Worried about cholesterol? Here's the thing… every cell membrane in your body is made up of fat and cholesterol. Your brain NEEDS cholesterol! Did you know the average person's liver makes 3,000 milligrams of cholesterol a day? In its natural, healthy, unstressed state your liver makes 75% of the cholesterol your body needs. The rest of the cholesterol that your body requires should come from the foods you eat. If we deprive ourselves of cholesterol, our liver overproduces cholesterol to make up the difference and stocks up. This process of stocking up can't shut off until you start eating cholesterol again. So, in reality a low fat, high carb diet can actually lead to heart dis-ease! The truth is, the biggest contributor to heart dis-ease risk is inflammation. When you're living the Keto lifestyle and are in the state of ketosis, you're getting rid of inflammation caused by sugar and high carb consumption. Coronary artery dis-ease occurs when a LDL particle (usually the small, dense one) in your bloodstream gets lodged in a lesion caused by inflammation in the artery wall. This is what causes the formation of the plaque that you hear about. If you have very low inflammation and no lesions for the LDL to get stuck in, your cholesterol numbers aren't really relevant. This subject is still a very hot topic in the medical community. We encourage you to please do your research and communicate with your physician. Ultimately you are in control of your health decisions.

Let's discuss BAD fats to AVOID at all costs! AVOID UNSATURATED AND HYDROGENATED FATS. They are POISON to your body! They cause chronic inflammation, weight gain, increased risks of cancer, autoimmune dis-ease and a multitude of other ailments that people suffer from. These oils are made from seeds and beans. The list of oils to avoid includes vegetable oil (there are absolutely NO VEGETABLES in vegetable oil), canola, safflower, cottonseed and soybean oil. Avoid these like the plague! They are not natural. You can't squeeze oil from seeds and beans! The oil has to be extracted with chemicals and processed in a factory. Yikes! Right!? You also need to avoid all fake fats like margarine. No brands mentioned, but if you can't believe it's not butter, it's not!!

Now that you know the good and bad fats let's look at what all those good fats are going to do for you. Fats make you feel full, they switch your body to fat burning and they eliminate inflammation to help your body heal just for starters. How awesome is that??

Sometimes it is a little difficult to get enough fats into your day so here is a super easy way to do it! BULLETPROOF COFFEE! It sounded really crazy at first and takes a little getting used to, but it is a great way to get in your fats. It is so good! Bulletproof coffee will keep you full for hours so here is the recipe to get you started. Pour fresh brewed coffee into a large coffee mug.

Add:

- 1 TBSP Butter (Grass-fed, non GMO, hormone free)
- 1 TBSP MCT oil or coconut oil
- Heavy Whipping Cream (to your liking)
- Liquid Stevia, Monkfruit or Erythritol to sweeten if preferred.
- Frothing it up using a battery operated mixer will create a fancy latte!

*Please note: We'll discuss sweeteners in a later chapter.

Proteins

You'll be eating a moderate amount of protein on this journey. Your protein intake will be 20-25% of your total daily intake of food. Our bodies do not store protein. If we consume more protein than our bodies use, the excess protein gets converted to glucose which could possibly raise your blood sugar, reduce ketones and in turn kick you out of ketosis and fat burning mode. This could also cause your insulin level to rise.

Even though you'll be eating a moderate amount of protein, it's vital for your body to survive. Protein sources contain essential amino acids and we can only get them from the foods we eat. Here's a really awesome fact: EGGS contain all 9 essential amino acids that our bodies need! There are endless ways to cook and eat them and hard boiled eggs are great to keep on hand when you need something quick to take on the go. The best protein sources are from organic, grass-fed fatty sources of meat so when you have a big juicy ribeye, slather it in butter and don't trim off the fat! When you have chicken, eat the dark meat with the skin on! Notice all the exclamation marks? This info really excites these southern born and raised girls for sure.

So, how do you find out the right amount of protein for you? The general thought is 1 gram of protein per 2.2 pounds of your weight. So, let's say you weigh 180 lbs. That would be about 80 grams of protein per day. For a person weighing 150 lbs., that would be about 68 grams per day. Here's the math: 1 ounce of protein is approximately 7 grams.

Carbs

What are carbs? The word "carb" is short for carbohydrate. The word "carb" is also synonymous with sugar and glucose so from here on out carbs, sugar and glucose will be used interchangeably but mostly referred to as carbs. You'll discover sugar comes in different forms and has lots of names that can be hidden to deceive and trip you up. That's why it's so important to read and understand labels and ingredients. The best rule of thumb is to stay away from foods that have labels. That is not realistic all the time, so we'll get into label reading a bit later in this book.

Your carb intake will be 5-10% (or less) of your total daily intake of food. Read this fact again…THERE ARE NO ESSENTIAL CARBS!! We have said it before but want to shout it once again because it's the truth! This is a REALLY hard concept to grasp because it is engrained into our brains all our lives that we need carbohydrates for a "balanced" diet. You have to have sides with all your meals, right?? No, you don't!

Angie: *"The fact that carbs aren't necessary went totally against everything I had learned in nursing school in my nutrition class and believe me, that was very little. Doctors have even less education on nutrition, go figure! When I'm sharing with family and friends, they want to argue this fact with me. You may be thinking I'm crazy too right about now but stay with me on this!"*

The Keto lifestyle focuses on very low carb consumption. As long as you are consuming a lot of carbs, your body will use the carbs for energy and will NOT burn fat. When you consume way more carbs than your body is burning it gets stored as body fat (especially in your belly, butt, and thighs) which leads to chronically high blood sugar levels and chronically high insulin levels. Every time you consume carbs it spikes both your blood sugar and your insulin levels making it impossible to burn the fat you have already stored.

The Keto lifestyle is also referred to as the LCHF (Low Carb, High Fat) way of life. Again, by low carb means you'll be eating 20 grams or less of carbs per day...that's really low compared to the amount of carbs the Standard American Diet says we should eat! SAD... perfect initials for the Standard American Diet don't you think?

Angie: *"I honestly thought the 20 grams of carbs amount was crazy at first because my diabetes dietician had recommended 165 grams of carbs a day for me as a type 1 diabetic! That's actually the American Diabetes Association's recommendations and just like the SAD recommendations, that's INSANITY! "*

Proteins and fats are essential but THERE ARE NO ESSENTIAL CARBS!

CHAPTER 6

The K.I.S.S. Method of Carb Counting and Label Reading

Should you count total or net Carbs? What's the difference? While it is always best to eat real foods, you know, the foods that don't have labels, reality says out of necessity we will be eating foods with labels pretty much every day to some extent. You'll find that some people will say you have to count total carbs and some who might argue that you need to count the net carbs. Do you subtract dietary fiber, sugar alcohols or both? What and who do you believe? Who is right? There are a lot of differing opinions and advice on both sides of the total or net carb debate. It can be quite confusing for you to figure out what you should do. Here's the great news…everyone agrees on the BASICS! So, we're going back to the basics and the K.I.S.S. method: KEEP CARBS LOW! That's it! That's as simple as it gets! You already know that your body will start to burn your stored body fat when you run out of carbs as a source of energy.

The debate is:

- How low should you go with your carb grams?
- Should you count total or net for fat loss to happen?

Clarity and confidence in your decision doesn't come from opinions, it comes from understanding the "whys". Once you understand the reasons why total and net carbs differ, you'll be able to figure out which way of counting works best and is right for you.

Let's look at a food label and define what total and net carbs are. Calculating total carbs on a food label is just the Total Carbohydrates grams listed. To calculate net carbs, you'll be subtracting Dietary Fiber and Sugar Alcohols (if any) from the Total Carbohydrates. Total Carbohydrate minus Dietary Fiber minus Sugar Alcohol (if any) = Net Carbs.

Total Carbohydrates (4 grams) - Dietary Fiber (1 gram) =
3 grams Net Carbs

* The total carbs for 2/3 cup from this package is 4 grams and net carbs is 3 grams.

Nutrition Facts

Serving Size 2/3 cup (85g)
Servings Per Container 5

Amount Per Serving	
Calories 25	
	% Daily Value*
Total Fat 0g	**0%**
Saturated Fat 0g	**0%**
Trans Fat 0g	
Cholesterol 0mg	**0%**
Sodium 25mg	**1%**
Total Carbohydrate 4g	**1%**
Dietary Fiber 1g	**4%**
Sugars 1g	
Protein 1g	**2%**

*Percent Daily Values are based on a 2,000 calorie diet

Let's explore the reasons why some people count total grams and some people count net grams. The truth is, both are right! Both ways work it's just we need to figure out which way works best for us as individuals.

Angie: *"If you're curious about how I personally count carbs, here's what I do. I focus on 20 grams of net carbs or less per day only because after I was diagnosed with type 1 diabetes and placed on an insulin pump, I was told that dietary fiber would not affect my blood sugar levels. I still count net carbs but have adjusted how many grams a day I consume. I keep my net carb grams way under 20 a day and some days I don't consume any carbs at all. You can adjust your carb amounts every day if you like."*

Reasons why some people count net carbs are because fiber isn't digested so it's believed to have little to no impact on blood sugar. Sugar alcohol doesn't increase blood sugar. Fiber and sugar alcohols have little to no effect on insulin levels.

Reasons why some people count total carbs are: People with metabolic issues like obesity and type 2 diabetes cannot tolerate carbs like others do. They have to count total or all carbs in order to lose weight especially the fiber that doesn't come from real, whole foods. There may be fiber in "low carb" snack bars or processed foods claiming to be Keto approved but the fiber they contain could possibly have an effect on blood sugar and ketone levels.

Then there's this thing called the "Cephalic Phase Insulin Response" where the mere taste of sweetness in your mouth can raise your insulin level! It's a REAL thing! Even if the sweet substance has zero carbs or calories, even if it doesn't raise your blood sugar and even if you just swish it around in your mouth and spit it out...it raises your insulin level!! Sugar alcohols can cause this response. That's another reason why people that count total carbs choose total carb counting instead of net.

The serving size and number of servings per container when reading a label is super important! When you look at the carb count, that's the number of carbs per serving. The label will not tell you the number of carbs in the whole container! But it will tell you how many servings in the container.

Nutrition Facts

Serving Size 1 oz (28g)
Servings Per Container 32

Amount Per Serving	
Calories 170	Calories from Fat 120
	% Daily Value*
Total Fat 13g	**20%**
Saturated Fat 2.5g	**13%**
Trans Fat 0g	
Cholesterol 0mg	**0%**
Sodium 120mg	**5%**
Total Carbohydrate 8g	**3%**
Dietary Fiber 1g	**4%**
Sugars 1g	
Protein 5g	**10%**

*Percent Daily Values are based on a 2,000 calorie diet.

Take this label as an example. You'll see that 1 ounce is 8 grams of total carbohydrates. Let's say this is a bag of cashews. If you measured out just one ounce, you're good. BUT, if you ate the whole container you'd blow it big time with 256 grams of total carbs!

Consider all the facts we've mentioned to choose whether you'll count total or net carbs then try the method that makes the most sense to you. You can start out with net and switch to total or vice versa. A word of advice would be to stick with one or the other until you get into ketosis. After you are in ketosis, feel free to tweak it until you find out what is right for you.

Bev: *"I have discovered that my body responds better with fewer carbs and that I really have to stay below 10 net carbs a day to keep my blood sugar down and my ketones up."*

So, how low can you go with carb grams? Most people start with 20 grams per day. You can go lower, but the general rule is not to go over 50 grams per day. As we've mentioned, you'll find there is so much advice and so many opinions that come from family, friends and even "experts" that can be truthful or flat out wrong. Here's the deal... it doesn't matter what worked for your friends or others, it doesn't even matter what the so-called experts say. At the end of the day all that matters is how your body responds and what works best for you!

Counting carbs and sticking to the limit is the most difficult part of changing your lifestyle but by far the most important for a lot of reasons. Once you've mastered this part you WILL NOT crave sugar like you did. Yes, that sounds crazy! Your taste buds will change, and you won't crave desserts or sweets like you did before. How is this possible? Are the Keto'ers who are saying this nuts? The fact is, it is REALLY TRUE! You will be able to sit happily chatting after a Keto meal while family and friends are indulging in desserts with millions of carbs and be able to resist the temptation. Ok, maybe that is a bit exaggerated... maybe 100-800 carbs, not millions but you get the idea!

Trust the process!
It may seem hard
before it becomes easy.

All this carb counting is going to be second nature to you after a couple weeks or so but in the beginning it's important to stick to your plan, be prepared, journal and have Keto friends. A great place to find Keto friends is on social media. We'll provide links to our Keto K.I.S.S. Facebook page, Instagram and website to stay connected on this journey in the back of this book.

CHAPTER 7

Carb Addiction, Keto Flu and Electrolytes

Let's talk about carb addiction. Uh oh! Yes, we are going there! It is a REAL thing. It can be ugly. Truth: Carb addiction may not be your fault, but IT IS YOUR PROBLEM! Mic drop! No apologies for that truth bomb because for most of us it's true and super hard to come to grips with. It's sad but what makes it even worse is that sugar is in just about everything, especially processed and fast foods. It's even hidden in things by the food industry that we would never imagine sugar would be in. Do you know why they do that? Because they know the power of sugar addiction and they know you will keep coming back for more! Reality says that we cannot completely get away from processed and fast foods with our busy lives. Sugar is in some very obvious places like soda, cookies and candy but it may not be as obvious in chips, bread, juices and even fruits or other foods. Even some veggies have more carbs than others. You are going to be pretty surprised at the incredibly high amounts of carbs in foods as you start this journey. It's really important to read the ingredients on labels and know the different names for sugar. Food manufacturers are required by the FDA to list the ingredients in order of their weight. The ingredient that weighs the most is listed first, and the ingredient listed last weighs the least. The take-away is to stay away from the foods where sugar is listed as one of the first 5 ingredients.

The unfortunate thing is, sugar has many different names and is hidden in almost every processed food there is! Of course, you will want to stay away from processed foods as much as possible, but what do you do when that is not possible in some situations? Sugar is hidden under more than 69 different names by the food industry. Let's look at where sugar hides and some of its aliases. Here's a list of the most common aliases: Sucrose, Dextrose, Fructose, Maltose, Lactose, Glucose, High Fructose Corn Syrup, Brown Rice Syrup, Maltodextrin, Molasses, Cane Juice, Fruit Juice Concentrate, Corn Sweetener, and Corn Syrup. For the most part any ingredient that isn't obviously sugar will typically end in the letters "-ose".

Honey, Maple Syrup and Agave come straight from nature and are considered to be super foods, nutrient dense and loaded with antioxidants. This may surprise you, but they are just SUGAR in liquid form! Ingesting them is just like eating sugar.

Then there's fruit. This is a sensitive subject for a lot of people. It's believed by some that fruits are the only source of certain vitamins and minerals and that fruits have fiber so they must be good for you. The truth is all fruits have a natural sugar called fructose and are really high in carbs. As an example, a banana has 24 grams of carbs and an apple has 19. Another truth is, there are plenty of the same vitamins and minerals in all kinds of leafy green vegetables that are low in carbs. You will notice there are fruits on the Keto K.I.S.S. Food List in the back of this book that you can enjoy occasionally. These are all berries... strawberries, blueberries, raspberries and blackberries.

The reason sugar is so addicting and why we struggle so much is because it stimulates dopamine, the feel-good, ecstasy hormone in our body. Studies show that a sugar addiction is more powerful than an addiction to cocaine! The more you consume, the more you want. Sugar is metabolized really quickly leaving you with some intense hunger. Since sugar is so addicting you may have some not so pleasant symptoms rear their ugly head in the beginning as you are eliminating it. We hate to mention stuff like this but to keep it real we must. You may have some of these symptoms: agitation, anxiety, headaches, insomnia, body aches and nausea, muscle cramps, and joint pain. While some may experience these symptoms, others may not. The good news is these should only be temporary.

There are two very important things to do to get past your sugar addiction, first is to have a SUPPORT SYSTEM in place and second, have a SOLID PLAN to stay on track. We have come to know over time how crucial and important it is to surround yourself with Keto buddies. It is great to have someone you can call or text when you need support or jump on our Facebook page and read through the posts to see how others have dealt with the same issues you are experiencing. You are not alone!

Surround yourself with Keto buddies.

To fight through carb addiction, it is important to clean out your kitchen of all temptations and to have Keto foods and snacks available. This is crucial. If you think you're going to really struggle, start your Keto lifestyle change slowly. Maybe start the first week or two by eliminating everything white and all beverages with sugar. Don't play games with yourself! If you're going to play games, you're only cheating yourself. Always purpose to do better today than you did yesterday.

If you've been reading about Keto or have friends or family doing Keto, you've probably heard the term "Keto Flu". First off, it's really not the flu but it may feel like you have the flu because of the similar symptoms. The best way to describe this process is your body is detoxing from carbs and carb addictions sort of like you're going through carb rehabilitation. You may or may not experience these physical symptoms, not everyone does. The symptoms may include headaches, feeling tired, constipation, diarrhea, muscle cramps, irritability, dizziness, and brain fog, all of which may be due to an electrolyte imbalance. It's important to keep your electrolytes in balance. If you do experience symptoms of Keto flu, please stay on track and know it's only temporary.

The 3 main electrolytes that you need to keep in check are sodium, potassium and magnesium. Sodium…you've got to have salt! It's vital and essential for life. You actually want to increase your intake of salt. Yes, that sounds crazy but here's why…when you're in ketosis your insulin level is lower and that's good, but insulin is also responsible for telling your kidneys to reabsorb sodium. Since your kidneys aren't getting the signal to reabsorb sodium, your kidneys flush salt out pretty fast. You need to quickly increase your salt intake to replenish what you're losing so your sodium level stays normal.

Potassium is a very important electrolyte for a lot of things but especially important for muscle contractions. If your potassium level is low, it could account for brain fog or even muscle aches and cramps. Avocados and green veggies are a good source of potassium.

Magnesium is another essential electrolyte. Magnesium is the regulator of pretty much every body system and is involved in every metabolic function in your body. If magnesium is low you could have symptoms like headaches, lightheadedness, dizziness, cramps and fatigue. To increase your magnesium level, you can eat green leafy vegetables, some nuts or avocados. As a reminder, Himalayan pink salt is a good source of minerals, electrolytes and magnesium. Some people decide to take magnesium supplements and that is totally ok.

If you happen to have any of the symptoms of Keto Flu, hang tight and stay the course. It's very temporary … that's a promise. There are a couple of popular sources of sodium, potassium and magnesium among Keto'ers that you might want to try. One is bone broth and the other is pickle juice. Yes, pickle juice! We'll just leave that one right there! <grins>

CHAPTER 8

Fasting, Intermittent Fasting, and the Huge Benefits That May Surprise You!

The BEST part of the Keto lifestyle is absolutely FREE! Yes, free! Fasting is the #1 form of detoxing your body from inflammation and toxins. It's a very important part of this Keto lifestyle. There are several really incredible benefits to fasting!! The biggest is the detoxing affect but here's a few more:

- Fat loss
- Lowers insulin levels
- Boosts your immune system
- Improves your mood
- Increases energy levels
- Turns off hunger

These next 3 benefits along with the benefits listed above are really amazing! They are autophagy, an increase in the human growth hormone and the creation of stem cells. Let's talk about each of these major benefits and then go into a couple of the most popular fasts on this Keto journey and how it's done.

Autophagy… an interesting word especially when you put the prefix and suffix together. You see, the word autophagy comes from the Greek words auto (self) and phagein (to eat). The thought of your body eating itself is just downright funny but that's exactly what it means! It's weirdly wonderful and it's actually pretty cool when you think about it. It's your body's way of getting rid of old, abnormal cell parts and replacing them with healthy new ones. Fun fact: Did you know your skin replaces itself every 35 days? All your new cells are made up of what you eat. You know the saying, "You are what you eat? It's true! So, how do you activate autophagy? You activate autophagy by fasting. The "sweet spot" for autophagy to really kick in seems to be after about 14 to 16 hours of fasting.

Fasting stimulates your body to produce Human Growth Hormone (HGH). You may be thinking, "I'm a grown adult. Why do I need human growth hormone??" Trust us, you NEED it! That's the hormone that will make all the brand-new cell parts to replace the old worn out ones when your body goes into autophagy! When you are fasting HGH levels skyrockets up incredibly high! This really benefits fat loss especially belly, butt and thighs. With all this going on, your insulin sensitivity improves making stored fat more accessible to be burned for energy.

Here is a really exciting thing about fasting…STEM CELLS! When you're fasting, your body starts to make stem cells. Stem cells go anywhere in your body to find injured body parts and repairs them! They can literally change and become any body part! In keeping this Keto lifestyle simple we will not go into stem cells here, but this is a subject that you might want to go deeper into because it's super fascinating. There's lots of incredible research being done in the area of stem cells.

Angie: *"I want to be upfront with the fact that I didn't fast for several months when I first started Keto mostly because I didn't understand all the benefits. Fasting sort of came natural after the first couple months or so because I really started listening to my body. I ate only when I felt hungry and stopped eating when I was satisfied. This turned into a natural fast and I didn't even realize I was doing it! When you're eating very low carb and high fat, you're not getting that huge blood sugar and insulin fluctuation that frequently makes you hungry. After learning all the wonderful benefits of fasting I did incorporate it on a daily basis. It's super easy once you're in ketosis."*

Fasting is the #1 form of detoxing your body from inflammation and toxins.

Bev: *"Recently, a friend of mine at work reminded me that when he first told me he was intermittent fasting that I looked at him like he had three heads. I actually thought he was crazy. Then, after lots of research I decided to try my first 16 hour fast. It has now become part of my routine and I love it. I make it a personal challenge to see if I can improve my blood sugar and ketone levels each time I fast."*

Fasting is something you can customize any way you want to. There are so many different ways to fast that you will find one that works for you. Not everyone fasts and there's no rule that says you must. Once you start this journey and get comfortable with it you may just find out that you are already naturally doing it!

On the Keto journey most people do what's called intermittent fasting (IF). Intermittent fasting is the most natural way to fast because of your circadian rhythm. Your circadian rhythm is a fancy word for your wake/sleep cycle. Your metabolism is sparked when daylight appears, and your body wakes up so IF is the perfect, natural way for your body to fast.

One thing that we would recommend before you start to fast is to get your carb addiction under control and be in ketosis first. Then when you first decide you want to start IF you may want to start off slow like maybe with a 12 hour fast. That would mean you'd go 12 hours not eating (including sleep time) and eat in a 12 hour window of time. You will find that is totally doable and pretty easy. You can start increasing your fasting time and decreasing your eating window time until you get to the 16/8 fast. The really cool benefits come around the 14 to 16 hour time of fasting. Most people do the 16/8 fast which seems to be the most comfortable for almost everyone. That means that you're fasting for 16 hours and eating in an 8 hour window of time. The 16 hours that you are fasting includes sleep time, of course! For example, start eating at 11 am and stop at 7 pm. If you do the 16/8 IF and follow our favorite rule, "Only eat when hungry, stop when satisfied", you will probably find that you are only eating 1 to 2 times a day! If you are just starting out or just considering this lifestyle you might think that sounds pretty crazy. Yeah, we did too!

Intermittent fasting (IF) can be done every day, several times a week or however often you choose. It's important to note that your digestive system needs rest to heal and recover. That's what fasting does!

You can drink water, tea (no sweeteners) and black coffee while you are fasting, nothing else. When you are coming out of your fast it's best to break your fast with fats and minimal protein. This will keep your blood sugar and insulin levels stable.

CHAPTER 9

TOXINS…Yikes!
Get Them Out of Your Life!

Here's a very vital topic that you REALLY need to understand and prioritize on your Keto journey! Please take everything in this chapter very seriously!

~ ANYTHING YOU PUT IN OR ON YOUR BODY HAS THE POTENTIAL TO BE THE SAFEST AND MOST POWERFUL MEDICINE OR THE SLOWEST FORM OF POISON. ~

Please pause, reread the statement above and let it sink in.

There's more to the Keto lifestyle and getting healthy than we realize. TOXINS ARE STORED IN YOUR BODY FAT! This is pretty shocking isn't it? Your body stores toxins in your fat as a defense mechanism.

Here's how that all works...

When your body is exposed to a large amount of toxins and can't safely get rid of them by natural detox pathways like your liver, the toxins are stored in your fat. When our livers are overburdened, we become sick and dis-ease sets in. Research has shown that a toxic overload can bypass liver processing and end up in your body fat. By storing toxins in your fat, your body is protecting your vital organs and tissues from damage. The danger and downside is ugly body fat, inflammation and serious health issues that could affect your heart and brain. If toxin exposure continues, the backlog continues to grow! Your liver has no way of really catching up. An overloaded liver won't release fat where toxins are stored no matter what you eat or how much you exercise. Toxins can actually cause weight gain in spite of all our dietary changes on this Keto journey. That's why it's so important to get rid of them! Stored toxins not only disrupt fat burning but also disrupts your hormones and endocrine system. The good news is that if you eliminate toxins, your liver and digestive system will heal. As your liver heals it can do its job of eliminating toxins again.

You're probably hearing more and more about the dangers of toxins and how they affect our lives on a daily basis. There are toxins in our personal care and cleaning products as well as in the processed foods we consume. You will most likely find that the way products are marketed, especially foods, makes it really tricky to find where toxins are hiding. It's super important to read labels and be aware of the most harmful ingredients. The guide to go by is simple.... if you can't pronounce it or don't recognize the ingredient, your body probably won't either! It's best to eat foods that don't have labels and use plant-based products for your household and personal care.

The most common toxins to avoid are:

- **Glyphosate** is a poisonous herbicide that's sprayed on plants (our food) and if you aren't eating organic, you're ingesting it.
- **Phthalates** are used to make plastics, makeup, lotions, air fresheners, and fragrances. It's a hormone disruptor!
- **Fluoride** is a neurotoxin and is toxic to our brain and nervous system!
- **Parabens** are food preservatives and are found in cosmetics. It's a hormone disruptor linked to cancer and reproductive disorders.
- **Bisphenol A (BPA)** is found in plastic water bottles. It mimics estrogen and disrupts hormones. It is linked to cancer, and heart and brain dis-ease.
- **Sodium Laurel Sulfate** is a foaming agent found in shampoos, soaps, and detergents. It is an endocrine disruptor, neurotoxin, causes organ toxicity, and linked to cancer.

This list goes on! There are literally thousands of toxins that are even approved and labeled as safe for us to use!

Toxins can actually cause weight gain in spite of all our dietary changes on this Keto journey.

Processed foods are full of toxins. The actual definition of a processed food is any food that is changed from its original form. Did you get that?? They are almost always full of carbs from lots of added sugar, the worst being high fructose corn syrup and artificial ingredients. Like we mentioned earlier, if you can't pronounce it or don't recognize an ingredient, your body won't either. Processed foods are engineered for overconsumption by the food industry! They want us addicted! The purpose is to keep you buying it with total disregard for your health and the health of your family.

The definition of a processed food is any food changed from its original form.

Once you know about toxins it's impossible to pretend it doesn't matter. It totally matters! The choices we make today WILL impact us tomorrow. With each passing day we lose some of the potential to regain our health. The pace at which our bodies degenerate is directly influenced by our DAILY CHOICES. By understanding the main causes of dis-ease and dysfunction, we can make dietary and lifestyle changes that promote health and a longer life. Who doesn't want that? So, to sum up toxins...eat organic, non-GMO, Keto foods without labels as much as possible. Use plant-based products in your home and detox your body by intermittent fasting or fasting for longer periods of time. Any positive change is a huge step in the right direction! Ditching and switching products to rid your home of toxins can be a process that takes time, but the results are powerful. You can never put a price on your family's health and wellness.

CHAPTER 10

KETOSIS!

How Do I Know I'm There?

First let's go over some things you might start to notice when you are entering ketosis.

- You may start to see your appetite decrease.
- You might notice you'll be able to go longer without feeling hungry.
- You'll probably notice you're sleeping better and wake up less groggy.
- A lot of people notice they're in a better mood… most of the time anyway!
- You'll begin to notice you have better focus and think more clearly.
- You'll have a steady energy level throughout the day without crashes.
- If you have experienced joint pain and inflammation, you'll

probably notice that going away.

- You may notice that you no longer have bloating, heartburn and reflux.
- You may notice a weird taste in your mouth.

Let's review what's happening. When you're in ketosis fat is leaving your cells and traveling to your liver to be changed into ketones to be used for energy. When you're making ketones, you can measure them. You seriously don't have to measure your ketones but it's kind of fun to know for sure, right? Some people are ok with seeing physical symptoms of ketosis while others want to use a test to know for sure. If you choose to test yourself, only test once or twice a week and don't stress out over it. Keep in mind that your ketones will fluctuate!

There are basically 3 types of tests for ketones: urine, breath and blood. The best time to test is in the morning before eating. Ketones fluctuate according to mealtimes, how hydrated you are, how much caffeine you've had, how much exercise you do and even your stress level.

The urine test is the cheapest but least accurate way of testing ketones. The urine test strips measure the amount of EXCESS ketones that you are producing. If your body isn't using all the ketones for energy, you just pee them out. The test results can really vary throughout the day. If you drink a lot of water, it can give you a false negative. The basic rule of thumb is if you get any shade of purple on the test strip you are in ketosis.

Let's talk about the breath test. These devices are called breathalyzers. You just blow into it for 20-30 seconds and get a reading. When you're burning ketones, you will be exhaling the byproduct of ketones called acetone. Don't freak out when you hear that! Yeah, it's acetone like the chemical found in nail polish remover but trust us, its ok! Your breath at this point could be described a number of ways like fruity, sweet, like nail polish, bruised or rotting apples or just plain rudely offensive. We promise the breath smell is only temporary! When your body adjusts to being in ketosis it will subside. The breathalyzers are pretty pricey at around $160.00 but you don't need to purchase any kind of strips to get results. The devices are a little more accurate than the urine strips, but they still have a high percentage of inaccuracy according to how you blow into it.

The most accurate ketone tester is the blood meter and of course it is the most expensive. The blood ketone meter measures the beta hydroxybutyrate (BHB) which is the fancy name for ketones in your bloodstream. The testing requires you to insert a test strip into the device, stick your finger for a small drop of blood and applying it to the strip to get the results. The test strips that you have to buy for the blood meter are a bit pricey.

When your body is
making ketones,
you can measure them.

CHAPTER 11

The Skinny on Sweeteners, and a Word About Alcohol

It's kind of ironic how when we start out on our Keto journeys that we look for sweeteners that are zero carbs to replace the sugar in the foods we're trying to eliminate. It's more of an endeavor to mimic the old way of eating rather than change anything because change is hard, right? That's totally understandable. Some of us can walk away from sugar with little or no struggles but let's be honest... most of us can't!

Even though there are some natural sweeteners and great recipes for sweet tasting foods and drinks available, there are some things we want you to consider before we talk about acceptable sweeteners and ones to avoid.

First of all, there's a potential to continue down a carb craving path. Keto friendly sweeteners are usually added to foods that closely mimic or replace the very foods that the Keto lifestyle gets rid of. This could promote mindless snacking and over-eating of these desserts and treats without paying attention to real hunger. The thing is, these treats do have carbs that must be counted. They can add up pretty quickly! These recipes could possibly keep you tied to old patterns of giving yourself sweet rewards that contributed to weight gain and dis-ease in the first place.

Here's the truth... ALL sweet tastes, whether real sugar or sugar substitutes, act on the same sweet taste receptors on your tongue. They can trigger similar brain pathways causing your body to maintain carb additions and cravings.

Any sweetener has the potential to stall or slow weight loss. There is information that suggests sweeteners in zero calorie beverages may cause long term weight gain and metabolic issues. It's best to always be cautious and conservative.

Even though it is best to avoid sweeteners if possible, we realize this just isn't always realistic! Birthdays, holidays, and events will come up in your life and there are ways to create special recipes to enjoy during these times with natural, zero carb sweeteners.

Please beware of hidden carbs in any sweeteners, even ones that are zero calories and zero carbs! The FDA allows products with 1 gram of carbs and less than 4 calories per serving to be labeled "zero calories and < 1 gram carbs". Always be aware of ingredients!

Here's what you've been waiting for... Let's talk about some Keto approved sweeteners!

STEVIA- It's from the leaves of the Stevia plant.

Positives:

- Zero calories, zero carbs
- No rise in insulin or blood sugar levels
- 200-350 times the sweetness of sugar

Negatives:

- Sweet but doesn't taste like sugar
- Many people complain about an aftertaste
- Hard to use in recipes

Comes in these forms: Liquid, Powder and Granulated

(Some granulated blends have Erythritol mixed in)

ERYTHRITOL- It's a sugar alcohol that occurs naturally in small quantities in some fruits. It is only partially absorbed and digested and could possibly cause some gastrointestinal discomfort in some people.

Positives:

- Zero calories, zero carbs
- No rise in insulin or blood sugar levels
- Easy to replace real sugar in recipes

Negatives:

- Doesn't "feel like" sugar in your mouth
- It has a cool sensation on your tongue
- Can cause bloating, gas, diarrhea

Comes in these forms: Granulated, Powdered Confectioner's and Granulated Brown.

MONKFRUIT- It is derived from a round, green fruit that grows in Southeast Asia. It was cultivated by monks hence the name.

Positives:

- It is 250 times the sweetness of sugar
- No rise in insulin or blood sugar levels
- It tastes good, most like sugar

- It doesn't cause digestive issues

Negatives:

- It's expensive
- Often mixed with fillers
- Comes in these forms: Granulated blends with Erythritol or Stevia, Pure Liquid Drops or Liquid Drops with Stevia

*Monkfruit is often mixed with Erythritol or Stevia to cut down on the expense and to improve its use in cooking.

XYLITOL- If you chew sugar-free gum, it is sweetened with Xylitol. It's the most common sweetener in sugar-free gum, toothpaste and mouthwashes. Like Erythritol, Xylitol is a sugar alcohol. Unlike Erythritol, Xylitol is only LOW CARB, not zero carb.

Positives:

- Tastes like sugar
- Only 50% is absorbed in small intestines
- Replaces sugar 1:1 in recipes

Negatives:

- May cause significant digestive upset
- Small amount of carbs can add up quickly

*May have a minor impact on insulin and blood sugar levels.

*PLEASE NOTE: Xylitol is HIGHLY TOXIC TO DOGS and other pets!! Even a small amount could possibly be fatal.

Any sweetener has the potential to stall or slow weight loss.

AVOID ALL ARTIFICIAL SWEETENERS!

You should especially avoid those that come in the pink, blue or yellow packets!! All artificial sweeteners have toxic side effects that aren't worth the risks. The side effects from these sweeteners include headaches, migraines, kidney damage, mood changes, depression, memory loss, vision problems, Attention Deficit Disorder, Alzheimer's and they are linked to cancer. The surprising side effects are worsening sugar addiction and causing weight gain instead of weight loss because of their toxic ingredients.

Artificial sweeteners are hidden in some very surprising and disturbing ways! These are products that have "Sugar-free" written on the labels. Look at the list of where they hide:

Toothpaste, mouthwash, children's chewable vitamins, cough syrup and liquid medicines, chewing gum, no-calorie waters and drinks, alcoholic beverages, frozen desserts, sugar-free candies, processed low carb snacks and many other places!

There are a few important things about sweeteners that we have discovered. We know we can all agree that we're all uniquely created. There's no 2 of us alike on this planet. Our body chemistries are all different as well as we all have things like emotions and habits that we deal with differently. We will handle sweeteners differently, too. Some of us may have reactions physically like an insulin/blood sugar response while others may only experience slight differences and there may be those who have no response at all. You will discover over time where you fit into this.

If you struggle with carb addiction, we really want to encourage you to avoid any desserts or treats, even the very low carb Keto recipes you will discover in the beginning! It's super important to deal with the issue of sugar addiction and get into your new lifestyle avoiding anything sweet for a while. We say that in love because we've been there. Even if the ingredients are Keto/low carb, it still can trigger both emotional and physical responses that could be very hard to navigate through on your journey.

Angie: *"I decided to avoid all the fruits that are Keto approved for a while in the beginning. Yes, that was hard, but it was very necessary for me. I added berries and Keto desserts back into my life after a couple of months and even then, not very often. That worked great for me. I couldn't believe how my taste buds changed and how I could totally walk away from some things I used to crave and overeat! Now that I've been on my Keto journey for quite some time, I can eat an occasional Keto dessert and treat without going crazy or over doing it. It's an amazing feeling to have conquered that in my life. It's all about your mindset and keeping your reason for beginning this journey ever before you."*

Bev: *"We are very different with our journeys. In the beginning, I had to eliminate all things sweet but as I continue on my journey, I have learned that my physical response to sweeteners has had a negative impact on my blood sugar and ketone levels. I scaled back on my use of sweeteners after several months when I became aware of the effect they had on me physically. "*

A WORD ABOUT ALCOHOL

Dry wines, both red and white, along with spirits are ok with the Keto lifestyle. You can mix spirits with a zero-carb mixer. Even though these are “ok”, it’s important to consider your liver has to stop and process alcohol as a toxin because basically that’s what alcohol is. Consuming alcohol may be hitting the pause button on fat burning during the time your liver is processing it. As far as we know it doesn’t kick you out of ketosis, but it can cause your inhibitions to be let down. If you’re tipsy you could possibly make poor choices that will certainly lead you to being kicked out of ketosis. It’s a good idea to just not consume alcohol at all if you’re prone to this.

CHAPTER 12

Detours, Pit Stops and Following Your Keto Map

On our journeys through life we've got to keep it real. There will be detours, potholes and maybe even an off-roading experience along the way. This is going to be true of your Keto lifestyle journey, too. The best way to handle these things is to look at them as learning experiences! It sometimes helps to throw in a little humor along the way too! What we love about this journey is you've got those who have gone before you and experienced some of the things you are going to come face to face with. Having said that, we're going to share some things we have learned traveling this path.

Your motivation for starting this journey is so important. The more intense your reason for changing your lifestyle, the more motivated you'll be. The more motivated you are, the faster you'll see changes and results that will excite you to stay the course. That's the point where you'll realize there's no turning back! If you haven't started Keto, here's the deal. We want you to commit to following this Keto lifestyle for at least 66 days. That means really stick with it and follow the Keto path closely for 66 days. If you don't like the changes you see, feel and experience you can go back to whatever you're currently doing. We put that out there because we're almost 100% sure you'll be thrilled with your results and never look back.

So, you've decided to jump onboard, let's get you ready for success! What's in your refrigerator and pantry? Uh oh! You should've seen ours in the beginning! CLEAN THEM OUT. Really! It's so important! Don't just make do with what you have now until you run out. Failing to plan is planning to fail! You will want to plan ahead by using the food list in the back of this book and in the accompanying journal. Customize your list and find the foods you love. If it's not on the list, it's a NO! It's really helpful to focus on all the things you CAN have rather than the things you need to avoid. Make it fun. There are so many wonderful Keto recipe books out there and of course Pinterest is great for finding yummy recipes. Always be cautious and really pay attention to the ingredients, serving size and macro counts of the recipes you find. It can get a bit tricky. The best advice is to stick with the foods that have no labels and create your own culinary masterpieces!

One more word about not keeping carb loaded foods in your frig and pantry...temptation and emotions can send you to the breaking point! THE STRUGGLE IS REAL! Not kidding! When you stock your kitchen, stock it up with Keto foods that you love, and you can grab quickly when you experience those intense moments. You'll be so glad you did!

Here's a tough one to tackle... cheat meals or days. Our advice is DON'T DO IT! We promise it's not worth it! Once you get into ketosis and start seeing miraculous results you won't want to.

Angie: *"I need to confess and be real for a moment. I seriously want to let you know I've struggled a time or two (maybe more). I can give you all the advice until I'm worn out, but I want you to learn from my slip-ups and poor decision making. Yes, it's the kind of lesson you learn quickly and don't forget. This dilemma came up at my son's wedding. I had choices but that evening I chose to go over my carb limit. UGH! I didn't sleep well that night and felt horrible the next day. Yucky things like bloating, being lethargic and generally blah both mentally and physically. The good news is when you're in ketosis for a while and should this ever happen to you, it's easy to jump right back in! I hope you don't ever experience this but if you do, don't be so hard on yourself and jump back onboard. Remember why you started and all the great things you're experiencing!"*

We think the best part of the Keto lifestyle is all the victories you get to celebrate all along the way! The majority of people we meet that are on the Keto journey start out to lose weight. We just want to emphasize again that it's so much more than losing weight! Here's the truth... the scale does not show the big picture. The scale is only a tool used to show just a small part of the fantastic things that are happening to your body.

The awesome things you're going to celebrate along the way are non-scale victories (NSV). What's a NSV? That's where you focus on all the other amazing things that you're noticing besides the weight loss. Sometimes the changes are not so noticeable but when you do actually notice them, you'll be "happy dancing" all over the place! Here are some questions you can ask yourself to make you more aware of non-scale victories:

- Are your clothes fitting differently?
- How's your focus? Are you squirreling less?
- How's your energy level? Is your afternoon slump gone?
- Are you sleeping better?
- How's your blood sugar or other labs?
- Are you feeling aches and pains less?
- Have your digestive issues pretty much gone away?
- How does your skin look and feel?
- How are your moods?
- Can you move your belt over a notch or 2?

Health isn't about the weight you lose. It's about the life you gain!

Non-scale victories are HUGE! Like the first time you go clothes shopping and find you need a smaller size, the day you realize you went through the whole day with lots of energy, the night you slept really well without bloating or heartburn and woke up refreshed… you get the idea! Let's be honest, when you look at the big picture, the NSV's are much more important than the scale numbers!

Ok, so we just addressed NSV's… now here's the kicker and the reason we had to talk about them…

THE SCALE IS A LIAR!

When you step on the scale it only tells you one thing. It tells you what your total body mass weighs. Your body mass includes your muscles, fat, amount of water, all of your organs, and bowel and bladder contents. The way the scale varies from day to day and even throughout the day is out of your control. The number on the scale depends on many factors and even the food you ate the day before could have an effect on today's weight. By the way, your body could possibly retain sometimes up to 5 pounds of fluid or more that could account for a weight gain. Just FYI, did you know that a gallon of water weighs 8 pounds?? That's just a random fact we thought we would add because that shocked us. Please keep in mind that FAT loss and WEIGHT loss are NOT the same thing!! Hear us out...weight and fat have very little in common. When we get on the scale, we automatically assume we've put on fat when it could be related to a lot of other factors. You could be retaining a little fluid or the steak you ate last night could be still be processing through your intestines!

If you're overly focused or obsessed with the number on the scale you will miss all the other miraculous changes that are happening in your body like all the NSV's we have mentioned. Our prayer is that you look beyond the scale at the big picture and get EXCITED!

We are going to keep it real as usual here. We have issues with the scale obsession thing and know many of you do also.

Bev: *"Early on I knew my clothes were fitting much differently so I knew my body was changing but, in my mind, I struggled with the scale numbers. I must admit, I EMOTIONALLY struggled with that as the scale is such a visual measurement of success for me. Even though I was feeling really great with positive changes like more energy and better focus, I fought with my emotions and the stronghold food had on me."*

Angie: *"I purposed from the beginning to weigh myself ONCE A WEEK instead of daily because I really struggled. I knew and admitted that I was obsessed and if I didn't see the number on the scale go down my stress level would go through the roof, especially if it went up!*

Mondays are my weight and measurement days. When I'm not seeing the scale move, I usually see a difference in my measurements. Even if it's just a 1/4-inch loss at least it's going in the right direction. If the scales don't move or my measurements don't change, I search for a NSV I can celebrate. I plot my weight on a graph and my version of a spreadsheet to help me stay on track. I actually look forward to Mondays!"

There's an awesome chart to record your weekly measurements in the Keto K.I.S.S. journal that you'll really love. However, you choose to track your weight and measurements, it's really exciting and awesome to look at your progress!

The scale should NEVER dictate your mood, emotions or set the tone for your day but we allow it to do that, don't we? Please let us encourage you to not give the scale that much power! If your main focus on your Keto journey is your overall health, then STOP focusing on the number you see on your scale. Yes, we're writing this to ourselves as well!

CHAPTER 13

Emotions and Mindless Eating ...the Struggle is REAL!

What if we told you that 90% of this Keto journey was emotional and mental and only 10% was physical?? It's absolutely TRUE! Your Keto journey will be more mental and emotional than physical. It's hard to believe or wrap your mind around this, isn't it? Most of us just focus on the physical aspect of learning what foods to eat and the things we need to do on the physical side but totally disregard our emotional struggles. It's not for lack of knowledge about what we should eat because most people get that part. There is a HUGE connection between our feelings, emotions and eating. This is especially true when you are endeavoring to change lifelong habits. We would do you a huge disservice to not address the emotional aspect of your lifestyle change since it involves 90% of your journey! That's why we chose to include this topic in our book and journal. We are confident in making this statement: Most diets fail because they fail to address the emotions, feelings and mental aspect of changing lifestyle habits. When you just focus on menu plans and recipes with instructions on how to follow them and disregard your thoughts and feelings, eventually you'll go back to your old habits. People get caught up with the busyness of day to day life and all the ups and downs of emotions and over time the old patterns just set back in. Don't misunderstand, these types of diets and weight loss programs do work for short periods of time. We're sure most of us could testify that the weight is lost initially but when we deviate or make a bad choice or two, we feel defeated and usually quit the plan which leads to packing the weight back on plus some. It's never a real lifestyle change, is it? How many times have we made that New Year's resolution, joined a gym or went on the latest fad diet with friends?

Most diets fail because they fail to address the emotional aspect of changing habits.

Most of us grew up in a culture where we suppressed our feelings and didn't ever share or talk about them. The expectation was, we were told to get over it, suck it up and deal with it and heaven forbid we'd cry! Did you ever hear, "Stop crying or I'll give you something to cry about!"?? A lot of us were also told that we needed to eat everything on our plates, too. We were expected to obey without question. If we made a mistake or didn't do as we were told it was followed by some sort of punishment usually leading to guilt and shame or some other negative emotion. All of these scenarios led to suppressed emotions and memories stored in our brains. We've coped with tucking our thoughts and feelings away from early childhood by putting on a facade and pretending everything was ok and never really talking about how we really felt inside. All these hurts and unfulfilled desires in our hearts lead to emotionally disconnecting.

Bev: *"Some of the negative things that have come from all those old internal messages buried in my subconscious are that food is the only comfort and support I have and that I just need to keep things to myself and be consoled by food. I sometimes wondered if I couldn't be perfect then why even try? These actions led to weighing over 300 pounds for over 30 years of my life! I became a type 2 diabetic, developed an autoimmune disease, have experienced joint issues that required surgeries, and was in counseling for over 2 years."*

It's been said that emotional eating can even start in the newborn period! Think about it, what do newborns do when they're hungry? They cry, right? If they are left to cry for long periods of time this sets up negative emotional pathways in their developing brains as early on as the newborn period. Did you know you can learn to redirect those negative actions into positive healthy outcomes for yourself even if they have been buried for decades? You really can! We're not in any way implying that this will be easy or quickly resolved.

Our emotions and mental health are something we will have to work on for the rest of our lives! There's no finish line or destination where you can proclaim that you are 100% emotionally healthy. It's all a part of your life's journey. When you are going through a lifestyle transformation of any kind, you need to be aware of your physical, mental, emotional and spiritual sides all at once. Does this seem a bit overwhelming? We can totally relate! But, if all these areas are not addressed, the Keto lifestyle will just be another diet that you go on for a short period of time and then go right back to where you started. Please let that sink in really good before we go on. Do you know what this does? It leaves you miserable, unfulfilled, with feelings of failure, more guilt and shame to reinforce all the other negative emotional pathways stored in your brain.

Without getting too nerdy, let's explore a little about your subconscious mind. It plays a big role in everything we feel and do and stores our experiences from very early in life. It is responsible for our behavior, emotions, thoughts and it handles 95% of what goes on in our mind while the conscious mind only handles about 5%. This was a surprising revelation! This helps explain something super important for you to know! Please hear and know this: regardless of how strong a desire or commitment we make to change a habit in our conscious mind, eventually the subconscious mind can win because of all the negative messages that are embedded in it! This is another thing you might need to read a few times for it really to sink in. Here's another way of putting this truth...A lot of the time it doesn't have anything to do with your lack of willpower but rather a consistent outpouring of all the negativity embedded in your subconscious. Wow! Did you really get that? Veering off the Keto path is most often not due to lack of willpower.

Emotional eating is defined as eating in response to your emotions and those emotions can be both negative and positive. While the term emotional eating often refers to eating as a means of coping with negative emotions, it also includes eating for positive emotions such as eating foods when you're celebrating an event or eating to enhance an already good mood. In all these situations, emotions are still driving your consumption of food. We often make light of our emotional eating and carb addiction by calling the foods we indulge in when stressed out as "comfort foods". The comfort foods we choose are pretty much always loaded with carbs. We usually grab foods like ice cream and pizza and would never even think about grabbing some veggies or a salad, right? Comfort foods are just that... they take us back to a time when we were happy, comfortable, safe and loved. Studies show that people reach for comfort foods when they feel isolated, alienated or alone.

Bev: *"Emotions weren't really expressed around our house as I was growing up. Instead of talking about emotions I was offered food. This is where I first learned of "comfort foods". I would hear things like, have some candy or how about some chips and dip? This is where the pattern began... food became my emotional comfort!"*

While it's certainly not easy to separate our emotions from our eating, it is crucial that we do! The first thing to remember is the fact that food's true purpose is to nourish our bodies. We need to get away from the words "comfort foods". That is really important. A great alternative to reaching for food for comfort is through visiting with friends, going for a walk, doing things we enjoy and engaging in other healthy activities.

Here are a few questions you can ask yourself. See how many of the following questions you answer "YES" to:

- Does stress or anxiety cause you to eat more?
- Do you eat even when you're not hungry?

- Does food soothe you when you are sad, mad, bored, anxious or any of the other feelings you face?
- Do you eat until you feel stuffed?
- Do you ever find yourself eating while doing other activities like watching TV or working on your computer?
- Does food make you feel comforted and safe?
- Do you feel as if food is your friend when you're lonely?
- Do you sometimes feel out of control and powerless around food?
- Do you feel the need to hide out when you eat or hide foods that you shouldn't be eating from others?
- Do you feel the need to eat even if you're not hungry at social gatherings?

The thing to remember above all else is food's purpose is for our body's nourishment and not a form of self-therapy. The great news though is there are ways to rewire these emotional pathways! The two very common negative emotions of guilt and shame have a tremendously powerful stronghold over most people. Once you learn that there is a way to break those chains of bondage, your life will be transformed in ways you never dreamed possible!

Read on....

CHAPTER 14

Mental Strongholds and Habits... Avoiding the Detours

We've already said that regardless of how strong a desire or commitment we make to change a habit in our conscious mind, eventually the subconscious mind can win because of all the negative messages that are embedded in it. There are a couple of words in that statement that we should talk about.

First is the word "desire". Our desire is when we are interested in something or basically, we want it. When we just desire something, we don't necessarily set a goal and take action to get the thing we desire or have interest in, it's just something we want. If the desire isn't strong enough to take action toward, we tend to make excuses and come up with reasons why we can't get it or maybe even blame others not really taking responsibility for really going for it. The other word is the word "commitment". When you make a commitment to yourself, you will do whatever it takes to let go of excuses and work toward goals you have set for yourself. The Keto lifestyle journey needs to be an "all in" lifelong commitment you make to yourself. Keep the words desire and commitment in mind as we're addressing mental strongholds and habits.

Let's go a little deeper…

Our brain can be rewired over time. Changing the way we think and act isn't always easy, but it is totally possible! We may have the desire to change our thoughts and actions and we may even succeed for short periods of time but ultimately, we fall back into our old patterns. A good example of this is all of those New Year's resolutions and diets we have started in the past. It seems that no matter how badly we want to change, either it doesn't happen for very long or doesn't happen at all. We're led to believe it's because we're weak or lack willpower. Research shows that it's not about willpower!

Think about your last diet, how long did it last? Why didn't it work? Let's look at the answer. Part of our brain wills us to do good. This is the CONSCIOUS part of our brain. The SUBCONSCIOUS part of our brain, where our emotions and memories are stored, is constantly directing most of our behavior.

Our conscious mind only handles 5% of what goes on in our lives on a daily basis while our subconscious mind handles the other 95%, as we have said. Not only does our subconscious mind control 95% of how we respond but it is super quick and can process INTERNAL and EXTERNAL things at the rate of 20 million per second! Our conscious mind can only process EXTERNAL things at the rate of 40 per second, way, way slower. This means by the time we're consciously aware of something happening, our subconscious is already processing it! Since our subconscious is so quick we most often react before we think. Have you ever said or done something before you really thought about it? Our subconscious minds can get us into trouble sometimes! So, what happens when our conscious mind wants to do something our subconscious mind doesn't want to do? Answer: Our subconscious mind will win the battle. That's why willpower only works for a short period of time.

Angie: *"Let me give you a recent example…Just today, my husband was walking to the kitchen and said, "I'm going to make some chicken salad. Do you want some?" My very first thought was, YES! I do! I got up and started to follow him to the kitchen but stopped in my tracks. NO! I can't eat his very yummy chicken salad right now because I had made the CONSCIOUS decision to fast today! My SUBCONSCIOUS mind really wanted to go for it. I could have justified eating the chicken salad by putting off fasting until tomorrow. I would have been upset with myself if I had done that though and only reinforced that negative feeling that is already well established in my brain. My decision was to stay the course, continue fasting and know that the reward (the yummy homemade chicken salad) would be there tomorrow!"*

Let's look at this in relation to your Keto lifestyle change. At the very beginning of our journey we're all in at 100%. We are determined and our conscious mind makes the commitment. We're really excited and can't wait to see the amazing transformations that we will be experiencing. Let's stop right there. Here's a spoiler alert that is important for you to grasp. Your subconscious mind was programed to see food as an emotional reward. Studies show it was almost completely programed by the time you were about 6 years old. Our brains are programed with both positive and negative emotions. The unfortunate thing is that we store more negative experiences than we do positive ones.

Bev: *"Early on I knew my clothes were fitting differently so I knew my body was changing but, in my mind, I struggled with the scale numbers. I must admit, I EMOTIONALLY struggled with that as the scale is such a visual measurement of success for me. Even though I was feeling really great with positive changes like more energy and better focus, I fought with my emotions and the stronghold food had on me."*

Here are some fascinating, nerdy things about your brain. We're keeping it simple, we promise. Your brain is made up of over 100 billion brain cells! All these brain cells communicate with each other. With the billions of brain cells that we have, there are over one thousand trillion possible connections between them. These connections are constantly changing. That just boggles your mind doesn't it?? While you're reading this right now, your brain cells are communicating with each other and changing their connective patterns to accommodate what you're reading.

For the sake of keeping this very deep subject simple, let's focus on the limbic portion of our brain as a whole even though it contains several parts. The limbic system is considered the subconscious part of our brain or some say it is the seat of our emotions, thoughts and memories. The limbic system is responsible for many things and is actually connected to our conscious brain. It communicates to our conscious brain our past experiences with fear, joy, disgust, anger, hurt and so many other emotions. There is a small part of the limbic system that is specifically connected to our ability to transform our minds and allows us to learn new things. That's great news!

Our conscious brain is the cortex. It deals with helping us regulate our emotions, complex thinking, creativity and language skills along with sensory and motor abilities. Our cortex or conscious brain makes us aware of who we are, makes decisions and has a lot to do with motivation and finding meaning in what we think and do.

We applaud you for hanging in there for this part, but we tried to keep it as simple as possible. Our brain is so fascinating and complicated beyond our comprehension. God's handiwork is so miraculous!

Here's what all the brain information was leading up to...our HABITS. Our habits have several parts. There's a CUE that triggers the habit, a REWARD that is associated with the cue and in between the cue and reward is the HABIT to reach the reward. So, it goes like this: cue > habit > reward. The motivator that drives the process is the craving for some need to be met. Keep in mind those cravings for emotional needs to be met goes way back to unmet needs and desires in our childhood.

The whole process with changing our old lifestyle is actually really simple. WE DID NOT SAY EASY! When you are changing old habits into new habits it creates new pathways in your brain! It may not come quickly, in fact, in reality it will take time to consciously build those new habits. IT TAKES A CONSCIOUS CHOICE. Remember, our conscious mind is slow; the subconscious is super quick and wins most of the battles. Real change is possible but here's the deal, this change will take discipline and a commitment. You are always just one decision away from a totally different life! You truly have to be serious about making this a lifestyle. Are you ready to make new neural pathways?

Let's go!

The keys to rewiring your brain and making those new pathways to change habits take these 2 things... CONSISTENCY and REPETITION. For real life change to happen, your new habits and mindset need to become part of your day to day life. You won't experience the power of a transformed life until you make a conscious decision to be consistent and repeating that changed habit. Get this...your Keto victories will be the result of your daily decisions! Small accomplishments every day builds confidence and feeds into your self-worth. Never underestimate the potential of these daily decisions to change your life.

Every day we have the opportunity to set ourselves up for success by choosing one simple, reoccurring habit in our daily life. We call it One Achievable Action or "OAA" for short. Simply pick out one OAA, write it down and be determined to accomplish it. Your OAA could be drinking 64 oz of water, not eating unless you are hungry, or putting all macros in your carb tracker. Whatever your daily OAA is, you'll discover at the end of the day how awesome it is to say to yourself "I did it"!

For real life change to happen, your new habits and mindset need to become part of your day to day life.

Journaling is a powerful tool that sets you up for a successful lifestyle change as well as future successes in your life. Journaling has the ability to help sort out our thoughts, feelings and emotions so you can process them and create lots of "ah-ha" moments.

Important things to journal are:

- Your OAA for the day
- Things you are grateful for
- Positive things in your day
- Things you learned
- Quiet time thoughts, meditation and prayer
- Specific feelings you're working through

Having daily specific goals and writing them in your journal is a solid way of making sure it gets done. If you haven't written your goal(s) on your daily "To Do" list, then you haven't set them! The power comes from verbalizing your goals either in conversation to someone or writing them down in your journal, either way it will help you stay accountable.

An attitude of gratitude is so vital in changing old habits. Gratitude is usually an overlooked or ignored part of creating new habits. The reason it is vital is because gratitude changes ALL your negative emotions! Think about it... when you are expressing gratitude you can't be worried, fearful, angry or experiencing any other negative emotion, right? Your emotions dictate your behavior so, driving the negative emotions away with gratefulness will change your life in wonderful ways! Make it a daily habit of writing down at least 3 things you are grateful for in your journal.

We can all agree that words are powerful. We underestimate the power of our words even though we believe they have power. Positive affirmations that are spoken out loud have the unbelievable power to change your life! Did you know your words can change you at the cellular level? It's scientifically proven! You can write words down to affirm your feeling and thoughts but there are miraculous benefits to speaking them out loud. Over time your positive affirmations spoken out loud change you whether you actually believe what you're saying at first or not. So, say those hard things!

- "I am beautiful"
- "I deserve to be healthy"
- "I am worthy of love"
- "I choose joy"
- "I am fearfully and wonderfully made"

If you find these affirmations difficult, say them every day anyway! If these positive affirmations aren't fitting what you would like to address or say, there are lots more affirmations out there to choose from. Seriously resolve to find your own affirmations to repeat every day.

Let's talk about relationships, community and the intense importance of Keto journey traveling companions. WE WERE CREATED FOR RELATIONSHIPS! That's the honest truth! When you are a part of a group of like-minded people incredible things happen! The encouragement, inspiration, support and things you learn from building relationships are truly priceless! Being a part of a Keto group of friends builds self-worth, trust, and is a safe place to share struggles as well as successes. The really awesome part is the accountability with love to help you stay on the Keto path. Nothing solidifies relationships like shared goals. When you are traveling the Keto journey with friends and are seeing victories it multiplies your joy! Being a part of a group of Keto journey friends that encourage you and cheer you on with their personal stories of success helps inspire you to keep stepping forward. You should never “Keto” alone!

*Our social media links are in the back of this book. Our heart’s desire is to create an awesome community with you! Please come join us!

You are always just one decision away from a totally different life!

CHAPTER 15

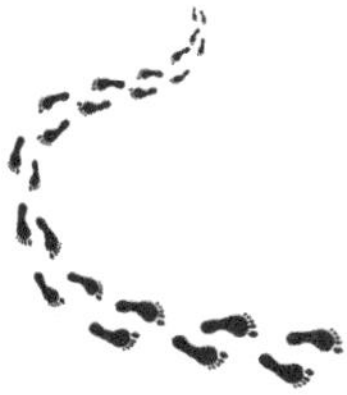

Aromatherapy: How Essential Oils Reroute Your GPS for a Successful Keto Journey

The role that aromatherapy with essential oils can play on your Keto journey is literally going to amaze and astonish you! Let's recap a couple things to start out... We've already talked about how our emotions are a powerful force that direct our thoughts, behaviors and actions. All these things are stored in the limbic system (subconscious) of our brains from a very early age. When you are on a journey that requires a lifestyle change, those old emotionally driven habits need to be changed and rerouted to positive pathways.

The choice to reroute your pathways is completely yours. We get to choose our own path but here's the dilemma with this, we're like travelers without a GPS. We just don't know how to get on the right path! Here's a HUGE revelation... we have an internal GPS; we're just not used to changing the input in it. Your GPS is your brain and you CAN change the input to guide you on this journey!

The connection between essential oils and rewiring your brain's pathways to change your emotional patterns is extraordinarily remarkable! Did you know that there is one outside (external) way to connect directly to the limbic system in your brain?? There is!! YOUR SENSE OF SMELL IS DIRECTLY CONNECTED TO THE LIMBIC SYSTEM OF YOUR BRAIN! Your sense of smell is the ONLY one of all your senses that is processed in this portion of your brain!

Smells have the ability to take us back to memories. Remember the pumpkin spice smell of fall, the smell of spruce or fir trees at Christmas, your grandmother's fresh baked cookies, and your mom's apple pie? Did you catch the food smell associations?? Memories in turn evoke certain emotions sometimes even before we're consciously aware of them. Research shows that in less than a second, a smell has the power to activate physical and emotional responses. Smells can instantly remind us of past events and can initiate either good or bad memories.

Research shows that in less than a second, a smell has the power to activate physical and emotional responses.

Your sense of smell is picked up by the olfactory bulb located inside of your nose. Get this…your olfactory bulb is not only relaying smells to your limbic system it is also relaying the things associated with the smells too! Your olfactory nerve cells are capable of learning and remembering information, but those cells are constantly changing and renewing! Every 6 to 10 weeks there are brand new olfactory neurons ready to take on new information and relay that new information to your limbic system as new messages! Here is an amazing fact to interject here…it's been said that the average time it takes to change a habit is about 66 days. So, if our olfactory nerve cells are renewing every 6 to 10 weeks, the timeframe just fits! We're sure by now you've noticed our excitement and a lot of exclamation points, that's because this information is so fascinating!

What does all of this have to do with aromatherapy and essential oils? To understand this powerful connection, we first need to know what essential oils are. Essential oils are the aromatic liquids found within shrubs, flowers, trees, roots, bushes, resins, rinds and seeds. Some people like to call essential oils "nature's living energy" because they contain unique constituents that provide a host of benefits for our health and wellness. Essential oils are made up of chemical constituents that are very small microscopic molecules. Once you breathe in an essential oil, thousands of microscopic molecules travel to your limbic system faster than the speed of light or sound through the olfactory bulb in your nose! MRI studies of the brain actually show how fast this happens! Just breathing in these molecules can soothe us, calm distress, restore memories, help us process trauma, increase confidence, boost courage and so much more all by interacting with our limbic system. Essential oils interact chemically and are carried to your limbic system via the olfactory bulb as new positive messages that you are creating or experiencing. These new, positive messages are replacing the old messages over time. Using essential oils can actually help you rewrite the way you think, feel and respond to situations!

It must be noted that casual and infrequent use of essential oils won't help change long term habits or patterns going on in your brain. Just using them every now and then won't get this rewiring response. When you really want to change the way you think, feel or act, rewriting your limiting beliefs or overcoming deeply ingrained emotions, you need a disciplined approach with CONSISTENCY and REPETITION. Using essential oils with the right tools like journaling, positive affirmations, prayer or other things you do in your daily personal development WILL transform your life!

Here are some tips and instructions on incorporating essential oils into your Keto lifestyle:

- Be consistent. You must be consistent because every thought or emotion you have reinforces the patterns (habits) that are already there. Carry your oils with you. Use them especially while praying, meditating or saying your positive affirmations out loud.
- Results take time. Using essential oils on a regular basis over time will produce the therapeutic results you are looking for. Remember olfactory nerve cells take 6 to 10 weeks to regenerate.
- Use essential oils specific to your needs for anything you may experience on this Keto lifestyle journey! Essential oils are incredibly versatile with a wide variety of uses due to their unique and complex chemical constituents. They have the ability to address many health and emotional issues that we face. By using essential oils, we are going back to our roots, literally. God gave us the earth when we were created, and we had everything we needed right from the beginning. After all essential oils and plants were mankind's first medicine.

IMPORTANT NOTE: It's very important to do your research on which company you get your oils from. There are many companies that will claim they have pure, 100% therapeutic, high quality essential oils.

The truth is, they can be adulterated and contain synthetic ingredients or may have been diluted. It is up to you to investigate and find the one you are comfortable with using for yourself and your family. Our suggestion is to look into how they are grown, harvested, distilled and what type of testing the company does. Do they have strict growing, harvesting and distilling guidelines? Can you go visit any of the farms at any time or do they keep secrets about how they run their company? Transparency is the key to finding a 100% therapeutic grade essential oils. The brand we use and the only one that we would ever recommend, meets all of the above criteria.

A few things about essential oil safety are:

- Never put essential oils in your eyes.
- Be cautious not to touch your eyes with your hands after applying essential oils.
- If an oil is "hot" or feels warm on your skin, you may add a carrier oil such as coconut oil to it.
- Don't apply any citrus oils to your skin if you are going to be out in the sun.

CHAPTER 16

Keto K.I.S.S. Essential Oil Blends

We are super excited to share with you the Keto K.I.S.S. Blends! After much prayer and direction, we were led to these specific combinations of essential oils that address real emotional struggles. We did a lot of experimenting and testing of these blends ourselves. THEY REALLY WORK! We developed 6 blends that we use on our Keto K.I.S.S. lifestyle journey. It is so incredible to see the gifts that God has given us from the beginning of time and all of the things that essential oils can do for us! We picked out single oils that address the following issues:

- Anger
- Anxiety
- Balances Blood Sugar
- Boosts Metabolism
- Boredom
- Concentration
- Confusion
- Curbs Appetite

- Frustration
- Grief
- Indecisiveness
- Moodiness
- Negativity
- Nervousness
- Occasional Depression
- Sadness
- Stress
- Worry

Each of our blends are made up of a combination of single oils and we want to introduce them to you individually before we discuss the blends. They are truly fascinating!

Bergamot belongs to the citrus family and has a fresh citrusy, sweet aroma that smells amazing when diffused or directly inhaled. It's used to reduce feelings of depression, anxiety, stress, agitation and nervous tension. It can help calm us when we are stressed and overwhelmed which can reduce our need to reach for comfort foods. Bergamot is at the top of our "go to" list of oils for emotional situations.

Cinnamon is an essential oil that's use goes back literally thousands of years. It is used as a powerful immune system booster as well as a blood sugar stabilizer. Cinnamon helps to decrease cravings and increase energy.

Clary Sage comes from the mint family and helps to balance estrogenic hormones. It has a very calming effect and can improve our sleep and dreams as well as reduce anxiety and fear.

Cypress essential oil is distilled from the needles and twigs of the tree. It aids the emotions during traumatic times and seasons of change. It can help us deal with grief, ease feelings of being overwhelmed, stimulate confidence, reduce guilt and perfectionism and support a sense of security.

Fennel has a very distinct smell and many properties that can aid in our healthy lifestyle journey. Sleep is a very important aspect of a healthy lifestyle and Fennel helps your body release its own natural melatonin so it can help with a good night's rest. It is also good for stabilizing blood sugar, increasing your metabolism and aids in helping your body convert fat to ketones to be used as energy.

Frankincense essential oil is mentioned in the Bible over 50 times. It is considered the holy anointing oil and was one of the gifts given to Jesus Christ at His birth. It was valued more than gold in ancient times and only the wealthy possessed it. Research has shown that the constituents stimulate the limbic system of the brain to help overcome occasional depression, anxiety, stress, and feelings of despair and hopelessness. Frankincense can increase spiritual awareness, promote meditation and uplift spirits. It is known to improve digestion and can affect our metabolic rate which can help with weight loss.

Geranium has a sweet floral, fresh, rose-like aroma. It is used for occasional depression, insomnia, nervous tension and stress. Geranium helps in releasing negative memories and balancing emotions. It fosters feelings of peace, well-being, and hope, along with establishing a sense of security. It also can help release toxins from within the liver and guess where the emotion anger is stored in your body… the liver!

Ginger essential oil is well known for supporting our digestive system but also helps regulate metabolism and reduces inflammation. It relieves anxiety, decreases nausea, and instills feelings of courage when inhaled.

Grapefruit essential oil is a refreshing and emotionally uplifting oil. Like other citrus essential oils, it is extracted through cold pressing the rind of the fruit. Grapefruit helps decrease stress and occasional depression. Its invigorating aroma can increase energy levels.

Lavender is an all-time favorite. Its aroma is so delightful, floral, yet woodsy and sweet. It has been said to be the "Swiss Army Knife" of essential oils due to its plethora of uses. It can soothe our nerves, lift our spirits, combat irritability, calm a panic attack, and can boost overall mental health. It is also known for its ability to lower cortisol levels, the stress hormone that makes our bodies hold on to excess fat. When we inhale this amazing oil through slow, deep breaths the aroma enters the limbic system of our brain. There it begins to decrease our anxiety and stress levels and may help to overcome the desire to emotionally overeat.

Lemon and ***Lime*** are both cold pressed from the rind and it takes approximately 75 rinds to make a 15 ml bottle of essential oil. Both oils are intense with a sharp, sweet, clean, citrusy aroma. They are both beneficial for anxiety, mental clarity, energy, improving memory, stress, and worry. Lemon and Lime can also help with insulin resistance and they are high in antioxidants. These amazing citrus oils have been found to improve clarify of thoughts with their invigorating fragrance. The detoxification properties if inhaled before meals can curb food cravings and help stop you from overeating while boosting your mood and improving your digestion.

Orange has such a fresh, fruity, sweet aroma that it can't help but make you smile when you smell it! It can relieve anxiety, curb your appetite, and is a powerful mood enhancer. Orange oil can have a sedative effect that helps with sleeping and relaxing.

Peppermint essential oil is a great oil to use for all thing's digestion related like nausea, indigestion, and heartburn. It is also used for calming, anger, headaches, fatigue, and as a breath freshener. The menthol in Peppermint can decrease your appetite and help reduce overeating. It stimulates the conscious mind by increasing mental accuracy by 28%.

Vetiver has a very heavy, earthy, smoky aroma. Its grounding, calming properties have proved helpful to relieving stress and shock from emotional traumas. It is a difficult oil to distill as it uses the root system of the plant. It is native to India and they refer to it as the "oil of tranquility". Vetiver is used to decrease anxiety and occasional depression.

Can a single drop of oil really do all that? We can assure you that they can! After using them for many years we could tell you story after story of all the ways our families use them every day and how they have literally changed our lives!

There are basically 3 ways to use essential oils… aromatically, topically and internally. We're only focusing on the AROMATIC, DIRECT INHALATION route in this book for addressing our emotions, feelings and moods. Direct inhalation is the fastest way to get essential oils into our bodies. When we're facing emotional situations that need a quick solution this is the best way!

Fascinating fact: It takes only a few seconds to get to the limbic system in our brains, 2 minutes to get into our blood stream and 20 minutes to reach every cell in our entire body! It really is that fast!

There are a few great ways to breathe in essential oils…

- Diffusing into the air with an ultrasonic essential oil diffuser.
- Placing a drop or 2 into the palm of your hands, rubbing them together, cupping them over your nose and slowly, deeply breathing them in.
- Using a nasal inhaler filled with the oils you choose holding it under one nostril at a time and breathing it in deeply while holding the other nostril closed. Repeat as many times as needed to get the effect you desire. For example, if you need to calm your anxiety, repeat with slow, deep breaths until you feel your body relaxing.

There's an amazing breathing technique that's taught in childbirth classes and various other situations where relaxation and emotional situations need to be addressed. Slow, methodical breathing using essential oils is powerful. Whether you are breathing your oils in from your cupped hands or using your nasal inhalers, you'll want to breathe slowly in through your nose and out through your mouth counting slowly to yourself… IN, two, three, four… OUT, two, three, four. You'll want to repeat this at least 6 times or as many times as you need to get the desired result you're looking for.

The following graphic shows you the issues that each of the KETO K.I.S.S. blends address as well as the recipes for making the nasal inhalers. Nasal inhalers are an easy, convenient way to carry your oils with you and you only need to refill them about once a month. You can also make these blends in a 15 ml bottle and we've provided the same "recipes" with the number of drops for the 15 ml bottles on the next page.

KETO KISS Essential Oil Blends Nasal Inhaler Recipes

Don't FREAK Out!

Anxiety, Fear, Stress, Worry

2 Clary Sage, 1 Frankincense, 2 Lemon, 2 Vetiver

Get Focused!

Concentration, Confusion, Indecisiveness, Nervousness

2 Frankincense, 4 Lime, 2 Geranium, 2 Lavender

No More Grumpy

Anger, Frustration, Moodiness, Negativity

2 Bergamot, 2 Clary Sage, 2 Lavender, 2 Peppermint

Feeling Fab

Anxiety, Boredom, Frustration, Stress

2 Bergamot, 2 Frankincense, 2 Lavender, 2 Lemon

Be Happy

Occasional Depression, Grief, Sadness

3 Bergamot, 1 Cypress, 1 Geranium, 1 Lavender, 2 Orange

Ready, Set...GO!

Curbs appetite, Balances blood sugar, Boosts metabolism

1 Ginger, 2 Peppermint, 1 Fennel, 1 Cinnamon Bark, 3 Grapefruit, 3 Lime

KETO KISS Essential Oil Blends 15 ml Bottle Recipes

Don't FREAK Out!

Anxiety, Fear, Stress, Worry

12 Clary Sage, 8 Frankincense,
12 Lemon, 12 Vetiver

Get Focused!

Concentration,
Confusion, Indecisiveness,
Nervousness

16 Frankincense, 24 Lime,
15 Geranium, 16 Lavender

No More Grumpy

Anger, Frustration,
Moodiness, Negativity

20 Bergamot, 20 Clary Sage,
20 Lavender, 20 Peppermint

Feeling Fab

Anxiety, Boredom,
Frustration, Stress

20 Bergamot, 20 Frankincense,
20 Lavender, 20 Lemon

Be Happy

Occasional Depression,
Grief, Sadness

15 Bergamot, 5 Cypress,
5 Geranium, 10 Lavender,
15 Orange

Ready, Set...GO!

Curbs appetite,
Balances blood sugar,
Boosts metabolism

15 Ginger, 30 Peppermint,
15 Fennel, 15 Cinnamon Bark,
30 Grapefruit, 30 Lime

You'll find that using these amazing essential oils blends on your Keto journey will not only change your emotions and moods on a daily basis, but will over time help change old habits into awesome new ones. Carry these blends with you everywhere. Here is a fun fact that you will love. If anyone close by is struggling with some emotions or moods that our Keto K.I.S.S. Blends address, you can nonchalantly help them out. For example, if they are feeling anxious, fearful, stressed or worried, grab your "Don't Freak Out" blend. If you have this blend mixed up into a 15 ml bottle simply drop a few drops into an essential oil diffuser or place a couple of drops into your hands, rub them together and fan them in the air. The really cool part is that you won't be the only one in the room experiencing the benefits! Everyone in the room will be positively affected. This is a huge game changer in your home, with your family or in your work environment!

CHAPTER 17

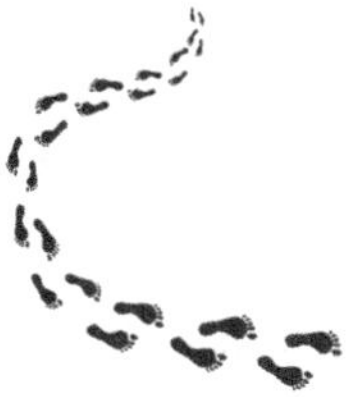

"STOP, THINK, & ACT!"

Steps to Successfully Change Habits

Our emotions and old messages can get in our way of successfully changing our habits. We created the **"STOP, THINK, & ACT!"** steps as a way to help us when times get tough. When our emotions are on the verge of getting out of control and we unconsciously find ourselves reaching for food, this is the time to apply the **"STOP, THINK, & ACT!"** steps.

Make a conscious effort to pause and take a 5-minute break. Set a timer if you need to but commit to sitting quietly for 5 minutes. Pausing is very important! Remember, your subconscious mind works way faster than your conscious mind. By pausing you are making a conscious decision and not a reactive one based on old ingrained emotional habits.

Following these **"STOP, THINK, & ACT!"** steps will help you create new pathways and habits.

- Grab your oil blends, a big glass of water, a pen and paper or your journal/planner.
- Find a quiet place to sit down and close your eyes and breathe in your oils deeply and slowly until you feel yourself begin to relax.
- Now have a conversation with yourself. Ask yourself the following questions while you continue to inhale your oils:
  - ~ Am I REALLY hungry?
  - ~ If I'm not really hungry, why do I want to eat?
  - ~ What emotions/feelings am I dealing with?
  - ~ Am I bored, stressed, anxious, overwhelmed?
  - ~ Do I just need a break from what I am doing?
  - ~ Is it a particular time of day that I usually eat?
- Jot down your answers and really think about them. Identifying cues that got you to this point. Becoming aware of what is going on is the key to changing old habits. Drink up that water!
- Next, think about what you could do instead of eating. Could you call a Keto friend? Work on a craft or project you enjoy? Take a walk? Read a book? Spend some time in prayer? Work in your yard or garden?

Note: We highly suggest you create a list of activities you enjoy ahead of time so you will be prepared!

Your subconscious mind works way faster than your conscious mind.

When you follow these steps consistently over time you will realize that you are learning to listen to your body's physical hunger cues instead of old emotional cues to eat. You will most likely find that you're not really hungry at all!

You may find too, that you just need to identify what it is that you are dealing with in your subconscious. This is something that we have to continually do on a daily basis, but we promise, it will get easier and you'll be amazed at what you learn about yourself.

CHAPTER 18

The K.I.S.S. List
Keeping It Super Simple!

The reason this book was written was to help you understand how incredibly SIMPLE the Keto lifestyle journey really is. Don't stress out or over complicate it! Have fun! Just focus on the basics... ALWAYS! So, without further ado, here's your....

K.I.S.S. List!

- Focus on keeping carb grams at 20 grams or less per day. That's it. Really!
- Eat only when hungry, stop when satisfied.
- Eat lots of good saturated fats.
- Eat a moderate amount of fatty sources of protein.
- Keep Keto snacks handy for those challenging times.
- Don't count calories... ever!

- If you veer off the path, get right back on track!
- Embrace intermittent fasting.
- Try to eat mostly foods without labels.
- Drink half your body weight in ounces of water every day.
- Take before/during/after photos for your testimony!
- Remember changing habits takes CONSISTENCY and REPETITION.
- Make sure to utilize the **"STOP, THINK, & ACT!"** steps.
- Carry your Keto K.I.S.S. Blends with you everywhere.
- Weigh and measure yourself only 1 time a week.
- Always plan ahead.
- Set realistic, measurable goals.
- Get moving even if it's just a walk every day.
- Don't Keto alone! Plug yourself into a Keto community.
- Go "Like" our Facebook page and join us on Instagram.
- Journal your journey in the Keto K.I.S.S. Journal every day.
- Celebrate ALL your non-scale victories!
- Develop a list of activities to celebrate your victories that does not include food like a mani/pedi, massage, take a walk, take a bath with essential oils, visit some friends, or play some music and dance!
- Focus on the things you can have, not things you have to avoid.
- Share this book and journal with your family and friends!
- Choose JOY and laugh a lot!

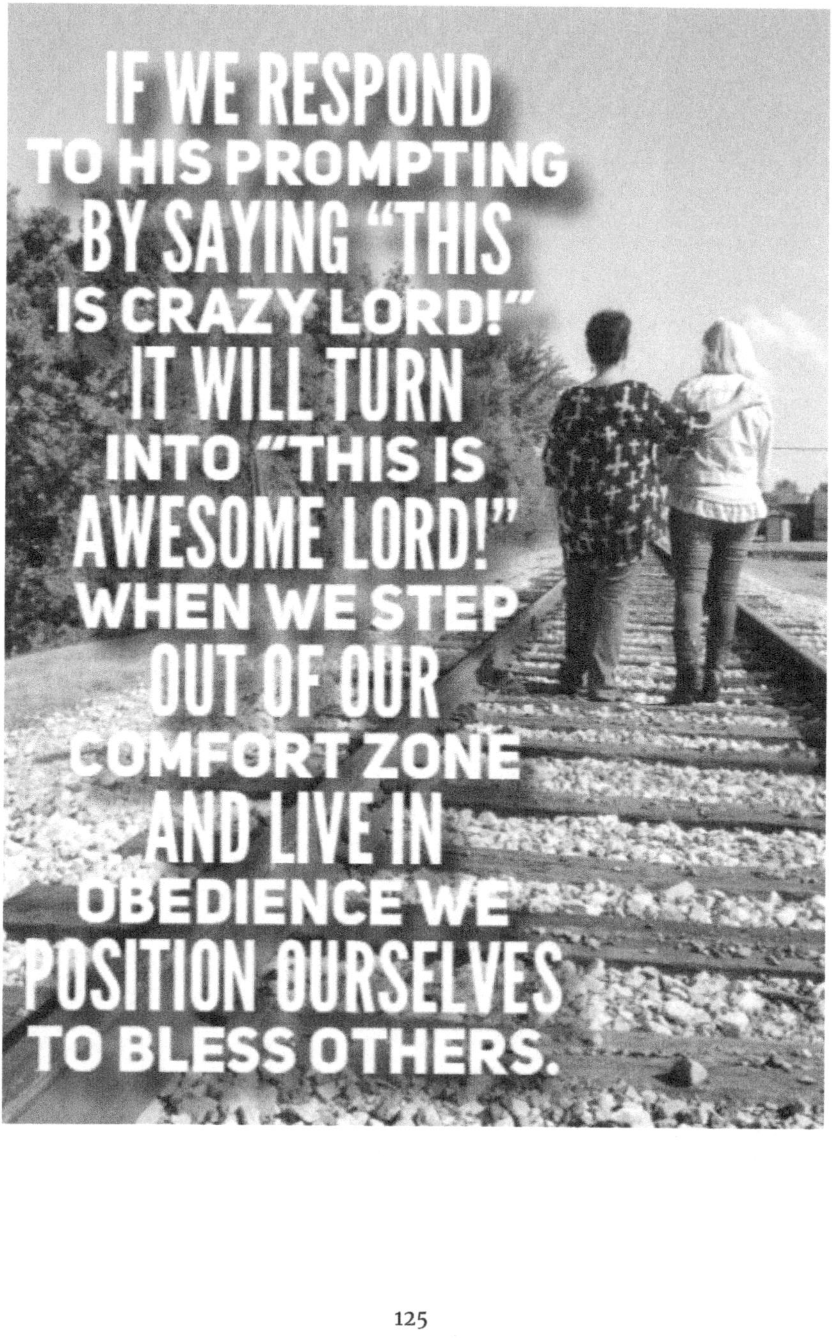
IF WE RESPOND
TO HIS PROMPTING
BY SAYING "THIS
IS CRAZY LORD!"
IT WILL TURN
INTO "THIS IS
AWESOME LORD!"
WHEN WE STEP
OUT OF OUR
COMFORT ZONE
AND LIVE IN
OBEDIENCE WE
POSITION OURSELVES
TO BLESS OTHERS.

APPENDIX

KETO KISS Food List

PROTEIN

Meat, Poultry, Eggs, Fish & Shellfish

- Beef: Ground beef, Steak, Ribs, Roast
- Pork: Bacon, Pork Chops, Ribs, Pork Loin, Sausage
- Poultry: Eggs, Chicken, Turkey, Duck, Goose, Cornish Hen, Quail
- Fish: Tuna, Salmon, Cod, Haddock, Halibut, Perch, Pollock, Sole, Tilapia, Trout, Flounder, Herring, Sardines, Anchovies
- Shellfish: Shrimp, Lobster, Clams, Oysters, Crab, Scallops, Squid
- Other: Pepperoni, Goat, Lamb, Veal, Venison

FATS

Oils, Fats, & Dairy

- Fats & Oils: Coconut Oil, Extra Virgin Olive Oil, MCT Oil, Avocado Oil, Almond Oil, , Sesame Oil, Flaxseed Oil, Macadamia Oil, Cod Liver Oil, Bacon or sausage grease, Ghee, Lard, Tallow
- Dairy: Grass Fed Butter, Heavy Whipping Cream, Cream Cheese, Cheese, String Cheese, Cottage Cheese, Sour Cream

BEVERAGES

- Water, Coffee, Black or Green Tea, Almond Milk, Coconut Milk, Macadamia Milk, Sparkling Water, Bone Broth, Broth, Stock

SWEETENERS

- Stevia, Erythritol, Monkfruit

KETO KISS Food List

PRODUCE

Vegetables

- Spinach, Spring mix, Kale, Romaine, Collard Greens, Zucchini, Spaghetti Squash, Green Beans, Eggplant, Cabbage, Brussels Sprouts, Broccoli, Asparagus, Cauliflower, Mushroom, Tomato, Onion, Cucumber, Radishes, Jalapeno Peppers, Banana Peppers, or Bell Peppers, Celery, Dill Pickles

Fruits

- Avocadoes, Lemons, Limes, Raspberries, Blueberries, Blackberries, Strawberries, Olives, 100% Cacao

NUTS & SEEDS

Nuts & Seeds

- Almond, Brazil, Coconut, Hazelnut, Macadamia, Pecan, Pine, Walnut Chia, Flax, Hemp, Pumpkin, Sesame, Sunflower

Flours & Nut Butters

- Almond, Brazil, Chia, Coconut, Flax, Hazelnut, Macadamia, Sunflower, Tahini

ENHANCEMENTS

Seasonings

- Himalayan Pink Salt, Black Pepper, Basil, Cayenne, Cinnamon, Cumin, Garlic Powder, Onion Powder, Paprika, Parsley, Red Pepper Flakes, Rosemary, Thyme, Turmeric

Condiments

- Ranch, Blue Cheese, Caesar, Italian Dressings, Aioli, Apple Cider Vinegar, Hot Sauce, Mayonnaise, Mustard, Soy Sauce, Wing Sauce, Pork Rinds

To Order Additional Books and Journals please visit our website at www.ketokisslifesle.com

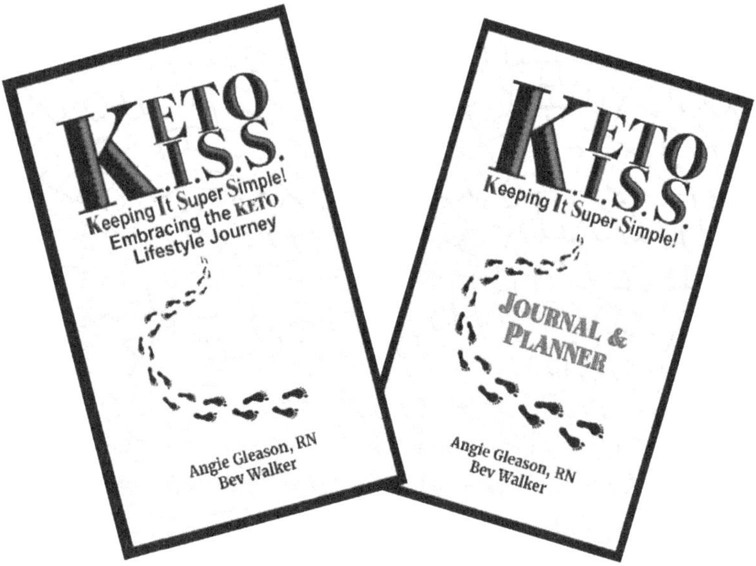

Ways to stay connected to us on your KETO K.I.S.S. Lifestyle Journey

WEBSITE:

www.ketokisslifestyle.com

SOCIAL MEDIA:

facebook.com/KETOKISSLifestyle

Instagram: ketokisslifestyle

EMAIL:

info@lifestylechangers.life